HEALTHY
WITHOUT HEALTH INSURANCE
PROTECT YOURSELF

MATTHEW EDLUND, M.D., M.O.H.

Other Books by Dr. Matthew Edlund

Psychological Time and Mental Illness

Gardner Press, 1987

The Body Clock Advantage

Adams Media/Circadian Press 2003

Designed to Last

Circadian Press 2010

The Power of Rest

Harper One 2010

FIRST EDITION

Library of Congress Cataloging-in-Publication Data is available upon request.

ISBN 978-0-9748927-1-9

CONTENTS

Preface and Acknowledgements

American health care may be on the brink of disaster, but a new health paradigm may just be starting its surge. Real health is complete physical, mental, social and spiritual well-being.

That's what people want – and are trying to get. It's one reason I wrote this book – so that you can find a way *on your own* to get healthy. But my real goal is to see this broader definition of health become applied to everyone.

Health should be the goal of health care.

And we can help reach that destination by looking at how human biology really works. We survive and thrive through regeneration. Human bodies – rather like communities – endlessly remake, renew and re-create themselves.

Our bodies work extraordinarily fast. The pumping proteins that let you read this sentence are made, used, repaired, destroyed and recycled in 60-90 minutes. Take away skeletal structures and *most of you is new* in a matter of weeks.

You want to take advantage of that fantastic opportunity – right now. Nothing stays the same – nothing. Get natural regeneration to work right and great goals can be achieved. Information rules the world. Whether it's software that a three-dimensional printer turns into a heart valve, or political ideas that explode the Middle East, information changes everything.

So it's time for us to do the same for health.

Regeneration works best by getting the body the right information – and information includes most everything we do. Information is much wider in scope than words, numbers, and texts. For example, food is a far larger source of body-changing information than the ingredients we read on a box.

Give the body the right information and it will regenerate properly. That means most of us should have a better shot at a long, vigorous life.

But it does not mean we will not get sick. As the Stoics wrote, we cannot change fate. Yet we can change our response to fate.

So people will get ill. Genetics and environment help determine whom, but a major factor is luck. Health care will always be necessary. But its goal should be health – not just for us as individuals, but for populations. And it should be applied in a manner that is fair, safe and cost-effective. Which means the current structure of the American "system" of health care needs to be thrown out the window.

We're stuck. You and I are going to have to do much of the heavy lifting ourselves – by ourselves. Fortunately, most of us can help regenerate our personal health – as well as the health of our communities. To do that we will need to use the right information – and apply it intelligently.

In some places that's already happened. Subpopulations in the U.S. are already living well into their nineties.

We can do it here.

Given our financial and political problems, we won't have much choice.

How Books Get Written

Whenever writing a book I find myself frequently thinking about my patients. I want them to feel good, to be excited about being alive.

They want me to cure their insomnia. Or make the pain in their big toe go away.

From those conversations I learn a lot. You find ways to get things to work. The body is almost infinitely resourceful. So is the human mind.

And people work collectively.

Einstein wrote about the "optical delusion" of human individuality. Even if you write alone in a remote mountain cabin, everything you pen is informed by the other seven billion "very unique" personalities living today – and the billions before.

We live in a sea of information – physical, social, mental. Anyone shaping that information is also shaped by it.

So I have way too many people to thank. Here are just a few: Professor Charles Edwards pointed to the work of Rudolf Schoenheimer in the 1930s describing the importance of recycling and regeneration. Tom Walker helped suggest the concept for this book – and much more. Janet Steckler and Jay Wilson were very helpful with ideas and editing, as were Professors Claudia and Glenn Cuomo and Suzanne and Gordon Stoltzner. Steve Reid, Bill and Sandie Herron gave useful advice, as did Mario Pietripaoli, Rosemarie Sette, George Valko and Jack Thompson.

I'm particularly grateful to my office manager, Mary LaPointe who's worked through some difficult circumstances, and my webmaster Dottie Rutledge. Dottie has been critically important to getting things done.

As for others who have helped, they're like the cells you see on a laboratory slide – too numerous to count.

Time Rules Life

This book was put together using what I thought was the best available current information.

Which can get blown away the next day.

Information always grows, always changes – just like we do. As a result I've put the references for this book on my two websites, wegethealthynow.com and therestdoctor.com.

They will change, too – as information changes.

So look for those references there – and the hundreds of articles I've written. Regeneration is much more than a biological event.

What we *think we know* changes – all the time.

Chapter 1 - Healthy Without Health Insurance

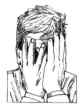

Health care is failing like housing, falling into confusion and collapse. It's one thing to be foreclosed on your home. It's another getting foreclosed from lifesaving treatment. As health care implodes you'll have to protect yourself. You need to do what you can to get healthy and feel healthy.

It's a good thing you can do that – simply and effectively.

The body regenerates itself quickly and powerfully. That regeneration constantly changes your body. It's never the same from day to day – even moment to moment. Learn to use your body the way it's built and most can live long and well.

Too many don't have any choice.

As of this writing, more than 50 million Americans have no version of health insurance. Nothing.

Fifty million are on Medicaid.

Many millions only possess "catastrophic" insurance.

Almost half the population can't afford to get ill.

American health care has failed you – and our country. Those with health insurance will see it pay for less and less – until even those "protected" cannot afford treatment required to survive.

Many of us need to get healthy, rapidly *and* cheaply. And you'll want to find a way to live that rejuvenates you and fills you with excitement at being alive.

And if you are sick, you want to get the health system to work for you – and not be worked over by the system.

It's time to get going. Fortunately, history is on your side.

Health Is the Goal of Health Care

Health is about how you live. Even when it does manage to function, American health care has far less impact on your life than lifestyle.

You want to put your health under *your* control.

A hundred years ago people died in their thirties. Nutrition, sanitation, education and vaccination doubled survival. Advances in medical care often did not add much more than a lick. Even antibiotics did relatively little to increase longevity.

What keeps you healthy is doing what your body is built to do – simple, practical, ordinary stuff. Actions produce results. What you do is what you become.

And you can do amazing things – particularly when you realize how much you *can* do. The longest-lived population in the world lives in the U.S. They're Asian American women in Suffolk County, N.Y. Eastern Long Island has the Hamptons, beaches, lovely clear bright skies – but is the landscape so unspeakably pleasant Asian American women should expect a lifespan of 95.6 years?

Or look at the 48,800 Asian American women in Bergen County, N.J. Northern New Jersey is studded with closed factories and chemical plants. It's a cancer hot spot. Yet those Bergen County women can expect to live 91.1 years – at least five years more than their mothers born overseas.

Do you hear much about America having the longest-lived people on earth? Or more about the love lives of the Kardashians?

Maybe you've figured out this story – that almost no one is making money encouraging the simple stuff that keeps you healthy. You'll hear much more about fad diets than about how your body really works.

Experts will argue, but putting together ordinary daily actions can add 10-15 years to your lifespan. Advanced medical care might – might add two to four years (and that last number is generous).

Maybe you don't care much about how long you'll last. Maybe you're just trying to get to work on time – or find work. Or perhaps your concern is juggling two crazily scheduled part-time jobs, taking care of the kids and paying the rent. And praying – praying you won't get the flu, which might cost you your income, your home and whatever insurance you've managed to hold.

Don't fear – the stuff that keeps you alive longer also helps keep you healthy and energetic. It can also make you happier, more productive – and looking better.

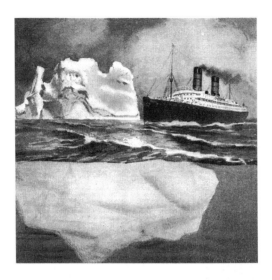

Our Titanic – The Amazing Business of Medicine

It's a fantastic, gigantic business. American health care itself is as large as the entire economy of France. Alone it would rank as the fifth single largest economy in the world – at least $2.6 trillion a year. It is as our politicians tell us, simply the best – beyond superlatives.

It's our Titanic.

Like the Titanic, it's bright and shiny and stuffed from stem to stern with the newest high-tech. It's got loads of folks in stratified levels above and below decks. It has gorgeous furniture, endless corridors and powerful publicists.

And our health care Titanic is heading for the ice floes – while the politicians and managers re-embroider the deck chairs.

Between 1960 and 1997 American health care costs rose 9.4% a year. They've continued to rocket faster than the growth rate of the economy.

Its product is always more of the same – more health care. Most industry leaders don't realize their product should be health – a long-living, productive, forward-seeing population. A nation where people look good and feel mentally and physically well.

Assuming present population increases and normal inflation, American health care costs should grow about 5% per year. That's at least a new $130 billion needed every year.

Where's the money going to come from?

Your pocket. Even if there's nothing more to pick. Until the whole system groans to a collapse.

And after that you'll probably be asked to pay much more.

According to the CIA, the U.S. presently ranks 50th in the world for life expectancy. Survival is certainly one measure of health quality. Our medical care is twice as costly per person as similarly developed countries, like Germany or Australia.

You can almost hear the cheerleader's cry – we're 50th! And we're twice the price!

Try being a salesman with a product that ranks 50th and costs twice as much as the competition.

Yet America's health care industry professes no such concerns selling its overpriced product. It fails to ever mention what countries learned a long time ago – **a healthy economy requires a healthy population.** And people's health is about lots of factors other than health care.

Plus there's virtually no incentive for the health insurance industry to keep you healthy. They'll tell you their contracts, especially with large corporations, change so fast they'd never get credit for improving people's future health.

Of course, that's not where they make their money. Their real profits come from increasing the overall size of that 2.6 trillion dollar U.S. health care pie. They take their share on every buck. And that is so, so much money that they can buy or block almost any politician in Washington or state houses they require – in order to keep the giant mess rolling along.

The whole point of insurance is that the fortunate pay for the unlucky. Risk factors matter, but there is always blind luck.

Nobody knows for sure which individual is going to get into a car wreck or be felled by heart disease – who will live and who will die.

But our political system has allowed the entire purpose of insurance to be stood on its head. Health insurers do not pool risk across the whole population. Instead, they cherry pick – only agreeing to insure you if you're not sick. Once you do get ill, you get to watch them try and dump you. Added health care costs may cause some employers to get rid of you. And if you are kept on, you may be forced to never leave a job you hate – because you believe you'll never get insured again.

Worse, future money for health care just isn't there. Employers are tired of paying for what Warren Buffett calls a tapeworm on the American economy. If the U.S. paid as much for its health care as Germany, we'd have more than $1 trillion free for other uses – lots of uses. Instead rates go up and coverage down – while the system goes off the rails.

The housing crisis helped blow up the world economy. It left millions without homes and tens of millions underwater on their mortgages. Millions never imagined they would know homelessness and hunger.

They know it now.

It's emotionally very hard for people when they can't pay the mortgage – and then lose their home. The emotional damage will be worse when people realize they can't afford treatment that keeps them alive.

The health care slow motion train wreck may take longer to crash than housing. Yet the effects may prove more devastating. Health care is at least 17% of the economy – far bigger than housing.

So you're stuck, folks. You're going to have to get healthy by yourselves. Given the state of the American economy, it's pretty much your patriotic duty.

Beating the Odds

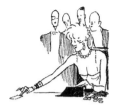

Following work teaching and researching in medical schools, I became a recovering academic. For the last 20 years I've practiced in economically shell-shocked Southwest Florida. Every week I watch my patients lose their jobs, their homes and their health insurance. Most of them ask me the same question – *what can I do now?*

Lots. That's why I'm writing this book – for you and for them. It's time to learn how to regenerate yourself. If that helps regenerate families, communities and the economy, so much the better.

Fate plays a large role in individual health. A 5-year-old can wake up with a bump on his leg. Next week his parents learn it's a sarcoma. You can be a quick sprinting 25-year-old vegetarian triathlete and still get run over by a confused 88-year-old on 10 different medications. Or you might change your ways like Eubie Blake, the great blues pianist who decided at age 96 that he enjoyed smoking so much he increased from two to three daily packs – and lasted out a century.

As doctors understand – and at the worst moments tell patients – life is a terminal disease. Even if you're Woody Allen and demand biological immortality, you will someday leave this life. But before you go you want to live on your own terms – fully alert and alive every second you've got.

So here's a second piece of medical advice – live this life like you've already gone through it once, and won't make the same mistakes. Except, you may ask, "since I haven't yet completely lived through this one, how do I know what mistakes to avoid?"

Because others have lived – lots of them. And enough people have studied what happened to those billions to give you a very good idea of what stuff you can do to live a healthy, rather happy long time.

Not that health advice is ever foolproof. Everything you learn in medical science has a shelf life – sometimes long, occasionally brutally short. In their first week of medical school students often hear a line supposedly uttered by a great 19th century physician, William Osler – "Fifty percent of what we're teaching you is right, and fifty percent is wrong. We just don't know which fifty percent."

Look at medical care in the last century and you'll quickly figure out what he was talking about.

Fortunately when it comes to getting and staying healthy, certain advice has stood the test of time.

They're basic ideas that combine into a system the simplest daily actions – how you eat; how you move; how you rest; how you socialize. The benefits, given their simplicity, are remarkable. You can:

- Get fewer colds
- Improve mood and decrease depression
- Improve immunity
- Avoid much heart disease, hypertension and stroke
- Help avoid many of the major cancers
- Control or lose weight
- Look better
- Feel far more alert
- And, yes, have a much bigger shot at living longer

Meanwhile, you'll be doing stuff that either costs little or nothing or plain *saves you money* – as well as your health.

And remember, health care is real expensive. Unlike bills you get from the grocery store or even your rent, medical costs leave most of us scratching our heads – and wondering if they added an extra zero to the charges. Make that two zeroes.

A single heart study you'll avoid might cost you $48,000 – or more. The ER work up for a painful tummy clocking in at $9,000 might have been avoided by standing after meals. Even that cut on your finger, which cost $3,200 – with the ER doc seeing you for all of 8.6 minutes – might not have happened if you had taken simple steps to correct your balance (these events were experienced by my patients).

Simple things work. They keep you alive. They save you money.

And they work because your body is mainly *new* – no matter what your age. Most of you is only about four weeks old.

That's because your body regenerates itself to survive – and thrive. Regeneration is how your body works.

It's not just health care that needs a different paradigm – so does health.

Your body is not a machine – it's an organism. An information processing organism where the work of life is fast and furious – so fast that most of you must quickly be replaced.

But *you're never replaced the same way.* Your body remakes itself, adapts and updates itself every moment you're alive. You see your hair grow; your nails grow – but not your brain. Or your heart. But they grow and develop – every second.

That they are continually remade provides you a fantastic opportunity.

Because you are made anew – remade constantly – you have the chance to replenish and remake your health and spirit. What you'll learn in this book are simple, ordinary activities you can take to remake and renew yourself. Do them and you can become healthier – and look, see and act in new ways. That's the promise of regeneration. It really helps having a simple guiding principle that can get – and keep you – healthy.

What This Book Is Not

Inevitably, there will be times you will get sick. Some illnesses you may muddle through with the support of family and friends. There are lots of books and articles on home remedies and do it yourself medical treatments. You may use those treatments when you can't access the crazy American health care system. But many times you will need the aid of a doctor and nurse.

Even if the health care system has forgotten its job is to keep people healthy, lots of individual health care workers chose their careers because they genuinely wanted to help people. Many work like dogs to care for people who cannot pay. Most communities have public clinics that will treat those without any cash, though quite a few don't advertise that fact. And by law hospitals must "stabilize" emergency cases, though many hospital administrators jump through hoops to violate the spirit and letter of those laws. Even if you walk into a "free" public hospital, you may walk out holding a bill you can't possibly pay.

So you want to find out what health care exists where you live that will not cost you your rent, your food money and what's left of your life savings. You need to know what you can do. Emergencies happen – routinely.

Expect them.

And plan for them. Even though how to get cheap, efficient medical care is a book in itself, I've added a short section on where you can go for health care – and what stuff to monitor in order to keep you healthy.

But remember – even if you possess "great" insurance, the American health care system is unsustainable. Old folks' health care costs a lot. And though the population is having fewer babies since the recession began in 2007, we're minting lots of old folks.

So no matter how old or young, it makes sense to learn what's necessary to live life fully – experiencing real health – through a few simple steps. You want to discover how to regenerate your body intelligently and inexpensively.

Which means first understanding why we get sick – the subject of the next chapter.

Summary

As the health care system falls apart you have to protect yourself. Some very simple steps can help you get real health – physical, mental, social and spiritual well-being. Those simple steps can help save you lots of money – even your life.

Chapter 2 - Why We Get Sick

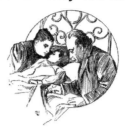

Blame Evolution

There's a pretty simple reason so many of us get sick and feel less happy and energetic than we should. We get ill – and often die – from preventable disease.

Blame evolution. Your human body evolved to survive terrifying, harsh conditions. Human genius, creativity and cooperation created an entirely different world.

Which happens to be the world we live in.

Your body was built for one world, but you live in another. Ironically, the world we created is one to which your body is unsuited.

A Disappearing Act

Humans have been on the Earth several million years. For most of that time we were struggling to survive.

Then about 75,000 years ago, we nearly didn't.

Human beings almost died out. Experts argue over how many of us were left, but we nearly starved to death. Those who survived migrated out to populate the world – and became the ancestors of most of us.

That's one reason why under the skin – despite our racial and ethnic differences – human beings are remarkably similar. The bodies we possess were built to survive horrific conditions. People with particularly effective immune systems survived incessant plagues. They lived long enough to regenerate and reproduce – and allow us to be born.

Throughout our evolution, food was really hard to find (for some of us it still is). So we became walking machines to get to it. We learned to cooperate in order to gather it. We managed to tweak our 30-foot gut and teeth so we could survive on tough, fibrous plants that were relatively plentiful, and still find and eat thousands of animals, insects and other creatures that were otherwise rare – or happy to escape us. Our metabolism flamed fast and furious as we foraged far and wide. We moved from ecosystem to ecosystem across the earth.

Then our brains got bigger and smarter. We created human civilization. Our species succeeded so well we dominate the planet.

Now our magnificent civilization is taking us over.

American Life

Doctors often wonder why people have devised so many different, ingenious and effective ways to destroy themselves.

And there's a simple answer. Lots of the stuff that destroys us is great fun – at least part of the time. And 21st century American life makes such fun a literal no-brainer.

Sometimes it almost seems that the American way of life was purposely designed to cause additional heart disease, stroke, cancer and depression.

But 21st century American life did not evolve in that fashion. It just took advantage of how evolution made us.

Vampires at the Blood Bank

We have bodies built through millions of years to eat almost anything, including grass (that's where grains come from). We survived chronic, intermittent starvation. Do we now need to spend untold hours going out to find food? Do we go through the hard labor of growing it ourselves?

No way. We drive to the supermarket. Almost everything we could possibly want to eat – and quite a lot else – *is all there.*

Plus, there's no need to lug it back home on your back. You've got a car to do that – or a bus or a train or a truck.

And you don't even need a friend to help you. You can carry all that fabulous stuff to your dwelling all on your own.

Once you're back home and finish eating, there are just so many amazing things to do. Night may fall but who wants to waste time with sleep? There's the Internet – virtually all of human knowledge and intelligence at your fingertips – including the latest, incredible shopping options. And there's television – hundreds of channels! Radio – hundreds of channels! There are movies from every country and every period. There's Twitter, and Facebook – the whole world to meet and greet; video games and multiplayer multilevel computer epics.

Why would you ever want to go to sleep?

So why are two thirds of Americans overweight? Why are we caricatured in the movie "WALL-E" as fat, snack-stomping couch potatoes so addicted to our electronic screens we don't know or care what's going on outside?

Because we have not yet heard the message – how little we need to know and do to effectively regenerate our bodies.

How You Get Healthy

The way our bodies are built got us into the mess we're in, the mess our tobacco, alcohol, food and drug companies so mercilessly exploit.

And our bodies will get us out of this mess.

The truth is that before we are unlucky enough or grow old enough to suffer chronic illness, we don't need to do that much to get healthy. We just have to know what are our bodies are built to do.

There's no need to go back to those nasty hunter-gatherer times. No need to go out into the wild to pick berries, dig grubs and chase insects. Once you know what to do, small changes should make the big difference.

Because small changes combine – and accumulate. Their actions add and then multiply. Before you notice it, you're different – in ways you might really, really like.

You just have to look at four basic actions in life – eating, moving, resting and socializing. Do smart things in one and you'll feel different. Do them together and you'll really feel different. Because making them work as a system really helps regenerate your tissues – and helps you experience real health.

You'll want to use this little book as a pocket guide to self-preservation and regeneration. Here are some benefits from doing the small stuff that fits how your body is built:

- It's enjoyable.
- You'll feel better.
- You'll look better.
- You'll become more energetic.
- It's cheap – often more inexpensive than how most people live – *and that's not including your savings on health care.*
- It gets you together with more people.
- You'll feel more fit and alive.
- It's ecologically sound.

In the phrase of Brooklynites, "what's not to like?"

You're about to find out. Let's start with one of the glories of life – food.

Summary

Want to know what causes disease in America? Blame evolution. Your body is simply not made for the perils and pleasures of 21st century America. But if you know how evolution made – and still remakes – your body, you can do the little that's needed to get and stay healthy. You then can use the knowledge of how your body regenerates as a simple guiding principle of what to do.

Chapter 3 – Eating

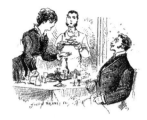

Ever suspect you were a vampire? With a few notable celebrity exceptions, probably not. Yet when we go to the supermarket, we're like vampires at the blood bank. And we often don't know how to stop ourselves from eating and eating and eating.

Is That Stuff Food, or an Addictive Drug?

Fast food is cheap – government subsidized cheap (your tax dollars). It's tasty. It's quick. It's available.

It also acts like a drug – an addictive drug.

My old office roommate at Bellevue, Dr. Nora Volkow, now head of the National Institute of Drug Abuse, once wrote grant proposals to see if foods acted in the brain in ways similar to addictive drugs. Nobody wanted to fund the research, but she found a way to do it.

What a difference the last few years have made. Here's what's presently acknowledged – and what you yourself should know –

• Foods filled with sugar and fat produce the same reward patterns in the brain as cocaine.

• Scan the brains of women who like to eat. Pictures of milkshakes light up the same place in the brain as addicts seeing their favorite drug.

• Give overweight young women sips of milkshakes. Scan their brains six months later. Those who gained weight show blunted responses in brain reward areas – just like drug addicts.

• Rats given sugar water or saccharinized water prefer it to cocaine.

• Rats allowed to drink soda-like drinks can't get enough. Block the effects of sugar – the rats develop tremors and shakes and other "drug" withdrawal symptoms.

When I ask patients who have tried both, most say they much prefer sugary sodas to cocaine.

So how do you beat this food trap?

Ask what your body is built to do.

Salt, Sugar, Fat and You

It's not amazing that we crave salt, sugar and fat. Just look at where we come from.

Salt, sugar and fat were not abundant through most of human evolution – not at all.

• Hunter-gatherer societies often fought over salt licks. Humans need perhaps 70-90 milligrams of salt a day to survive.

• Average American daily intake – 3300 to 4000 mg. About 50 times what we need. Yet take salt away from a chef and witness a dying restaurant. For many of us no salt means no taste.

And what do the brain and red blood cells survive on? Sugar – in the form of glucose. You have to starve for a week before you can use fat to replace sugar. Every morning you wake up you're digesting your muscle proteins to provide that sugar – one reason breakfast is the most important meal of the day.

Fat is also something we cannot live without. Your brain is mostly fat. The wondrously elastic lining of your cells is filled with fat.

Without certain, sometimes hard to obtain essential fatty acids, you die.

No wonder ice cream is the perfect food. It's a spectacular confection of salt, sugar and fat – and with the industrial ingenuity of the American food industry, loads of added artificial sweeteners, flavors and texture improving preservatives.

Which is one reason I've priced the eBook version of this text for less than your average ice cream cone.

What Should I Eat? The Mayan Food Pyramid

The U.S. Department of Agriculture likes to put out new food pyramids every decade or so. Good stuff to eat is placed at the broad base of the pyramid. Bad stuff goes on the little edges of the tippy top.

It's sad the USDA didn't consider that the original and most impressive pyramids – the Egyptian ones – were staggeringly expensive repositories for the dead.

Yet Americans are now habituated to putting their dietary components into some type of food pyramid. So instead of an Egyptian pyramid we'll use a Mayan pyramid.

Mayan pyramids were mostly made up of a base. There's no point on their tops.

They cut off pretty shortly above their base. Instead, on their highest surface, stood a flat altar used for religious ceremonies. Many Mayan religious rituals required human sacrifice.

And that's what lots of processed foods deserve – the executioner's axe. Though some can be pardoned for special occasions like birthdays, New Year's and Christmas, or just used in small amounts for brief, intense pleasures.

What kinds of food live at the base of our pyramid? Foods that have been studied more extensively than others and have long been consumed. Since individual foods are amazingly complex, they're also foods that work together as cuisines. Here's the group inside the pyramid –

- Vegetables
- Fruits
- Cereals
- Nuts
- Fish
- Foods that are also useful drugs – teas and coffee

What lies on the top of our Mayan food pyramid? Everything else. Particularly most processed food.

Meat does not make the list because it takes about eight pounds of grain to make one pound of beef – a huge environmental, energy and ecological cost to the present and future. And fatty meats are implicated in heart disease, stroke, cancers and perhaps autoimmune disease.

Does that mean you shouldn't eat meat? No. It just means you shouldn't eat huge amounts of it. Because meat is sadly expensive to your environment and your pocketbook – even if it tastes great.

It just makes sense to use meat as a condiment rather than the main energy source. It's better to enjoy the taste without the associated health trouble.

Yogurt and dairy products are a two-way street, with nice effects regarding some nutrients and varied effects on gut bacteria, allergy and immunity as we age. Dairy products can be used with less worry in younger populations. Fish makes the cut not because of our stellar wastefulness in how we harvest fish – about 90% of many of our favorite fish stocks have already disappeared from the sea. It's because some fishes remain abundant and inexpensive, and because fish fat appears to be healthy for our brains and arteries. Sixty percent of your brain is fat.

Despite what you've been taught – or may think – most of us are fatheads.

Simple Rules to Eat

Michael Pollan has written some very smart rules for eating. He's even written a short, highly useful book made up entirely of food rules.

So here's one rule most of you can follow:

Eat Plants. Lots of plants. Whole plants.

It's really time for you to enjoy using your 30-foot gut – and to have that 30-foot gut enjoy you.

Because there's more than your own cells down there – there's about 100 trillion bacteria. Together they have at least 150 times the number of individual genes than humans possess. We certainly need our bacteria to digest and process our food – they create a third of the detritus produced when digestion is over.

They also change our immunity and help manage our overall health. Treat your bacteria right and they'll treat you right.

Which according to the present results of research, means less autoimmune diseases like asthma or ulcerative colitis. Easier weight control. Even, perhaps, an ability to combat stress and experience much better mood – lactobacilli do that for mice. Give lactobacilli (found in yogurt) to mice and they are much harder to stress and get depressed. So putting the right plants into your daily food should make your bacteria very happy with you.

So what can we eat that's cheap and good?

Cheap Eats – Vegetables for Less Than a Buck Per Pound

Here's a short list:

Kale – I get a giant bunch of the stuff for $1.99 and it lasts six or seven different servings; useful cold or cooked. Lots of fascinating chemicals inside; supposedly helps cut back on macular degeneration, the increasingly common scourge of the old.

Celery – fiber that works to move the gut, filled with dozens of chemicals that should convince your brain there's lots of food – so you don't have to eat so much. It's useful for those who prefer to eat more than three meals a day.

Sweet Potatoes – One patient goes to her favorite market on Saturday and bargains, from three for a dollar to four for a dollar. I usually see it at around 40 cents a pound. Lots of cool stuff inside, including varied and complicated fats and proteins – and that's just the very few ingredients that have been studied.

(**Note** - those who suffer from kidney stones may want to give kale, celery and sweet potato a miss. And please, carefully wash all vegetables and fruits before eating.)

Lentils – I go to the Middle Eastern store and buy their dried version for about $2 a pound; Publix versions go for a buck and a half, Internet options for less. Soak it in water and it mushrooms into the equivalent of five or six entrees; cookable with almost any flavors, and often best when slowly simmered and liberally spiced. Cans of the stuff are generally about $1.29 to 1.49 at this writing, for 14 ounces.

Fava Beans – about the same price as lentils, and cooked in similar ways; multiple entrees per pound, and easy to put together with other vegetables; high, like other beans, in protein, and very different kinds of fat; perhaps originally got popular because of its effects in helping avoid malaria.

Black Eyed Peas – high in protein, easy to cook, cheap and widely available.

Green Peas – cheap, high in protein, easy to cook.

Carrots – good to eat cold or hot, and with much more than carotenoids inside. When it comes to food, as with clothing, **color can be good for you** – and makes you feel good, too.

There are dozens of other vegetables – virtually all of them are good for you, particularly in combination. They just cost a bit more – except when they're in season.

Or when you know how to buy them.

How to Buy Food

1. Go to markets – fresher produce coupled with generally cheaper prices. Friends of mine who live in Paris and other expensive cities say they could not survive without shopping at markets. Fresh foods also have more useful, easier to digest ingredients.

2. Buy in bulk. What works for Walmart also works for you – it's a lot cheaper buying 25 pounds of oats than one pound. Come home with a shopping bag containing at least four different vegetables – like pinto beans, kale, carrots, lentils – and four different fruits – like oranges, apples, bananas and plums (especially in season – see below).

3. Exchange with friends. Some may love lentils, while you just want a few. Some prefer a little taste of kale in a salad; others love to cook large bunches of the stuff.

4. Don't avoid frozen vegetables – or cans. Not all inner city groceries have lots of cheap, fresh produce. There are problems with cans – bisphenol A, or BPA, linked to birth defects, is added to many metal can linings. Sadly most foods canned or wrapped in the U.S. add loads of salt and not infrequently sugar or high fructose corn syrup (HFCS).

Who would have thought herring in wine sauce would be stuffed with high fructose corn syrup? I didn't.

That said, you could strain canned vegetables of their added salt and sugar. And canned foods can last a while, be quickly available for emergencies, and provide what is often a cheaper alternative for some very useful foods. And these days money is tight.

Cheap Eats – Fruits for Less than a Buck Per Pound:

Apples – yes, they've got alar, unless they're truly organic. They've often been pressed and gassed and frozen for a year. Yet they are cheap, good for your teeth, and filled with some very good things – many such "white" foods can prevent strokes. They're useful snacks and desserts – a great way to polish off a meal and your teeth at the same time.

Bananas – lots of potassium, packed with many minerals and vitamins amidst the sugary core. They are also cheap.

Oranges – a bright, useful color to spice up your plate, whether it's in the form of this fruit – or from a carrot or pumpkin.

Lots of different fruits – pears, apricots, kiwi, lemons, and berries – all possess their own advantages. They're just not as cheap as apples or bananas, except when they're in season or better, locally grown.

Fruits may contain much fructose, but their advantages are multiple. When it comes to healthy eating, color is the spice of life.

Put Five Colors on Your Plate

The Japanese smoke like fiends. It's good business for the Treasury – tobacco is a government monopoly and a huge funding source. Japanese work ferociously long days. After work, salarymen often have to pack themselves into dingy bars and listen to their bosses for hours – before commuting home drunk to arrive after midnight. Women's economic advancement is so blocked and home life so stultifying that many go on marriage strike – which still doesn't help get them a leg up in management. For Japanese females, joining a corporate board is considered a miracle. Japan's population is rapidly shrinking, their population quickly aging, and their main island has been blasted by the tsunami/nuclear catastrophe at Fukushima.

And the Japanese live longer than the people of any other nation – well into their eighties.

There are many reasons why the Japanese live so long. One reason is their deep and protective social connections. Another cause for their longevity is how they eat – many different kinds of foods in innumerable combinations.

Nutritional variety is a hallmark of other long-lived, healthy populations.

The Japanese say that the healthy way to eat is to put five colors on your plate. They're not talking about fruit loops or gaily decorated bean curd. They mean different colors made up of many different natural foods.

Which means different types of fiber. Protein. Vitamins. Minerals. Carbohydrates. Spices.

Plus the many other thousands of substances in foods that have not been well studied or characterized but nevertheless do much to help us control weight and keep us well. Talking about protein, carbohydrate and fat does not even begin to suggest the richness, complexity and usefulness of food information.

So when it comes healthy eating, variety really helps. And if you allow that different shades of green can count as different colors, putting five colors into a meal becomes a lot easier than it first sounds. **When you eat, think color.**

Cheap Whole Cereals

Rolled oats – generally less than a buck per pound. Can be cooked or eaten raw. Besides enormous amounts of fiber, oats produce micelles – fat trappers that can quickly lower your cholesterol. Oats also have lots of protein and can be added to almost any cereal.

The Roman Army lived off oats. They're not just for horses.

Rye flakes – not as cheap as oats, but tasty, and good for protein and fiber.

Buckwheat – easy to cook, simple to buy.

Steel cut oat groats – cheap and very, very fibrous. Very useful for those whose guts feel too slow.

NOTE on BREAKFAST CEREALS ***

Many of America's "favorite foods" – cereals sold on shelves with brightly colored packaging – are really concoctions of industrially simplified grains. Unhappily, they are usually stripped of their fibrous coverings and protein-filled cores. The starchy remainder is then packaged together with lots of salt, sugar, and fat – plus artificial flavorings and preservatives that belong back in the bottom of the oil barrel. Not only are such store-bought cereals less healthy than whole grains, they're generally a whole lot more expensive. Often store-bought cereals are less grains than a kind of cookie or dessert (check if honey, HFCS, cane sugar or similar "sugar equivalents" is the first or second ingredient). Read labels carefully before adding breakfast cereals to your larder. That includes the granolas sold in whole food stores, which contain some mighty nice ingredients amidst the added cane sugar and HFCS.

Many people take raw whole grains and make their own granolas.

Nuts

Nuts are not cheap – with the exception of soy nuts and peanuts. Yet they are deeply varied, densely caloric food groups all on their own. Like cereals, nuts are seeds – and seeds have more calories than leaves, a big issue if you want to control weight.

That's because the brain often interprets bulk as food. Put a lot of fibrous vegetables into the beginning of a meal, and people may eat 300-400 less calories per day.

Fiber can fill you up, and make you eat less.

That said, nuts are often highly nutritious, easy to carry, and very easy to eat. They're particularly convenient foods for those who like consuming more than three meals to control weight or diabetes.

Research-favored nuts at present include:

Walnuts – chunky, tasty, crunchy, and good at lowering cholesterol and heart disease risk.

 Almonds – not necessarily as healthy overall as walnuts, but not much worse, either. Definitely a good add on to other meals. *Nutritional variety is healthy in itself.*

Cheap Fish

As you move up the fish food chain you find more fish that eat other fish – which means more mercury. Mercury is tasteless, but the less of it you ingest the better. Which is a really good reason to stick with small fishes with lots of fatty oils like:

Sardines – cheap, and not yet globally overfished.

Herring – a global staple for millennia.

Tuna – cheap in the standard canned variety – if not as delicious as the disappearing blue fin beloved of sushi fanciers. Contains a bit too much mercury for many, especially pregnant women.

Salmon – healthy when wild. Still has similar problems to tuna.

Canned fish have their problems – besides BPA. But if you play your cards right, you can get healthy fish for around $4-$5 bucks a pound. Wild Alaskan salmon, packed whole in cans, is a relative steal.

And a little bit goes a long way. Getting two to three ounces of fish a day can be plenty – lots of protein, fatty oils, and vitamins. Fish also goes well with salads of all kinds, especially those containing many different vegetables.

When To Eat

Breakfast:

If at all possible, eat breakfast for several reasons:

1. **To control weight**.

When you wake in the morning you're in starvation mode. You're cutting up muscle protein to get required glucose for your brain and red blood cells.

People who eat breakfast have a much better chance of losing weight.

Parents who eat breakfast have kids with better weight control.

Eat one meal a day at breakfast and you'll lose weight; eat the same meal at night and you'll gain.

You metabolize food in about half the time in the morning than the evening.

You've got more insulin available in the morning than later.

2. **For energy**.

You need the fuel and materials in the morning.

And you can add coffee or black and green teas to:

Wake you UP

Decrease your risk of diabetes

Decrease your chance of Parkinsonism

Perhaps lower your chances of some tumors, like prostate cancer.

Half of American dietary anti-oxidants now come from coffee. Fortunately, now you've learned about lots of other cheap, abundant foods that can get and keep you healthy.

Plus recognize that foods contain much more than the proteins, carbohydrates and fats beloved of nutritionists. Recent studies show different plant foods literally push MicroRNAs into your gut – stuff that directly changes gene expression. One MicroRNA we get from eating rice rapidly shifts cholesterol levels.

The information in food is extremely complex. That's why you need to eat lots of different foods – not one "superfood" at a time.

What to Eat for Breakfast:

Lots of different stuff – consider getting those five colors together. You can combine oats, rye flakes, fruits, nuts – with varied kinds of milks. Here you can mix processed milks – varying from skim milk, to soymilk, almond milk and rice milk. Generally, the more varied the ingredients, the tastier your meal can be.

Make breakfast the biggest meal of your day – or simply a bigger meal than the usual pop tart – and you'll have a much better shot at controlling your size and waistline. That includes controlling the amount of unhealthy fat surrounding your gut organs – called visceral fat.

Because you really want to avoid **TOFI** – Thin Outside, Fat Inside. Many young women are now developing diabetes – even when they're thin. That's because visceral fat is an endocrine gland that can set you up for heart disease, stroke, and inflammation. Visceral fat develops quickly with the traditional high sugar, high fat American diet – and can lie beneath a truly narrow exterior. So please don't envy models who live on sugar and coffee. Nutritional variety can really help prevent TOFI – as can moving around (see the next chapter).

Lunch

Try for a colorful meal – filled with several brightly colored "superfoods" the media so loves to tout. Lunch is a great time for salads. If you want to have a dessert, make it a whole fruit like apples, kiwi or pears. Mix, match and mate together many different foods for the best taste and healthy results.

Dinner

Make it small if possible. Dinners are excellent times for social eating – a good time to talk about what's in food, where it comes from, and how it's prepared with children, family and friends.

The same meal eaten at dinner – compared with morning – will produce higher glucose and lipid levels. That's not good for your mid-section or your arteries.

Lots of varied cooked vegetables can be very filling at dinner, and keep you healthy as well.

Snacks

If you can run a disciplined five or six meals a day diet, more power to you. If you can't, then snacking is not your way to get and stay healthy. If you can't stop intermittent snacking, try first drinking a large cup of water and strolling five minutes before you eat – *and walk for a longer time after.*

If you must use snack please think of these "snack foods:"

- Celery
- Apples
- Carrots
- Small amounts of nuts – like less than what fits in your palm.

Avoid the "fun for you foods" marketed by Pepsi and other giant processed food producers – even the new "reduced fat" versions. They're an improvement over what existed before – which is not saying much.

Natural is better. **And cheaper.**

Where To Eat

Eat at home – with friends and family – when you can. You'll have a much better idea of what you're eating and how much.

You'll also be better able to control cost.

Restaurants

If you're a reasonably normal human you crave salt, sugar, and fat in your food. That's what restaurants will give you – in spades.

Not to mention loads of flavorings, preservatives and condiments that originate in petrochemical plants.

Don't expect the chefs to know where everything comes from. They may know where the animals were raised – but not how they were raised. The additives in spices – forget that. Chefs' interests are different. They're trying to make meals really tasty – so you'll come back.

There's a simple way to make restaurants work – tell them exactly what you want.

You can ask for steamed vegetables – or grilled vegetables. Put a small piece of fish on the side – or specify how you want a whole fish cooked. Perhaps add a few shaved nuts.

Or request a salad with all sorts of ingredients you desire – like sardines or tofu, Brussels sprouts or broccoli.

If you don't feel you can tell the chef what to cook – and most restaurants these days are used to taking directions – ask that their standard dishes be modified.

Dressings can go on the side. You can ask that no mayonnaise go into the sushi. Turn down the offered banana cakes and bread in a basket.

In restaurants it pays to take control. You'll feel empowered, plus know more about what's really going into your gut. You are much more than you eat – especially when you **specify what you'll eat.**

And try different foods so you can learn from restaurants what you like to eat. If you can cook it yourself – even partially – you might save a bundle. A restaurant meal foregone might pay for several days of food you cook yourself.

Booze

It's strange to recognize that wine, beer, and spirits – which help cause dozens of different tumors plus brain, heart, liver, lung and kidney damage – can actually be good for you.

But they can. The trick is to treat them for what they are – legal drugs.

Alcohol is a carcinogen. But most drugs have their uses. Alcohol can help keep arteries open, and in some people, perhaps even prevent Alzheimer's.

The trick – use alcohol in small, steady doses. One glass of wine three of four times a week, or up to one glass a day in women and two in men may produce healthy effects – beyond the many lethal ones. For some adults, coronary artery disease risk can plummet 30%.

Too much booze and you're in trouble, though. Use alcohol the way it's meant to be used – for conviviality, personal calm, and social engagement.

In other words, use it sparingly. **Drugs can prove addictive – not just food.**

High Fructose Corn Syrup, Sugar and Starch

The sugar industry would like you to believe that sugar is just sugar. They'll tell you it doesn't matter that it comes from beets, sugar cane, or giant vats of industrially processed corn.

Please be skeptical:

• Sugar itself may eventually prove to be pro-inflammatory. Most times your body has more than enough inflammation without adding more sources.

• Sugar may be addictive. It certainly acts as an appetite enhancer. Just like in the children's book "The Phantom Tollbooth," you can eat a whole meal, follow it with dessert and become hungry all over again.

• In adolescents and adults HFCS provokes visceral fat creation – and pre-diabetic conditions.

• Starches are basically sugar polymers. Get that piece of white bread into the gut and before you know it, gut enzymes have transformed it into a big wad of sugar. Perhaps 30-35% of sugar will change into fat, much of it inside your abdomen.

You're still better off eating whole grains and vegetables than you are eating most processed starches – including bread. Most breads contain large amounts of salt. Whole natural foods are usually more complex inside – and often cheaper.

Vitamins

Recent studies demonstrate that daily vitamins – particularly in older women – may be worse than useless. In older, Midwestern women, added vitamins increased the risk of death.

Different groups need different vitamins. Most kids need a lot – as do pregnant and nursing women.

The jury is still out on vitamin D. The National Institute of Medicine thinks adding vitamin D may increase cancer risk and overall mortality for many in the population. Vitamin D researchers disagree vigorously.

Calcium is a similar story. Some people who add calcium to the diet – which Americans do to an almost unprecedented degree – seem to increase the calcification of coronary arteries. Yet other studies claim added calcium improves overall survival.

Bottom line – you'll get most all of the vitamins you want by eating whole foods – especially whole plant foods. Variety adds more than spice to life – vitamins and minerals come along, too, especially with colorful foods.

Summary

Foods are amazingly complex. Each food can contain thousands of different, potentially healthy substances. Common foods even contain genetic material that will immediately change your gene expression.

Yet knowing how to eat them can be simple:

Eat whole foods – particularly plants.

Adopt a Mayan food pyramid – with vegetables, fruits, cereals, nuts, fish, tea and coffee found at the base – and everything else placed sparingly on the flat top.

Eat breakfast to control weight – but avoid store bought breakfast cereals that are desserts in disguise.

Avoid getting TOFI – thin on the outside, fat on the inside. Abdominal fat is a hormonal gland that works against you.

Use booze as a drug and it can help you.

Get restaurants to give you exactly what you want – you're paying.

It's best to think about food – not just eat it. Ask yourself the regeneration question. Is what I'm eating helping my body regenerate – or making it more difficult?

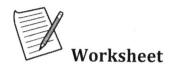

Worksheet

Your body uses up an enormous amount of material and fuel in a day. Give it the right stuff and it has a much easier time rebuilding itself. Regeneration is extremely rapid. Most of your heart, for example, is replaced and remade inside three days.

Yes, *life is fast.*

Every human body is unique, with its own requirements for proper regeneration. Still, most of us can benefit from a few simple suggestions. So here's a worksheet for your food day:

Start with breakfast. Hippocrates was right – it's critical to health (unless you're a shift worker and can't live according to a normal day-night schedule).

Think of eating cereals – mixed and combined cereals. Each food has hundreds or thousands of different ingredients. **Nutritional variety means you get more of the good stuff.**

Put together whole oats with other grains – like rye flakes. Add multi-grain granolas for nutritional variety – and for taste. Watch out for sugar, though. Lots of granolas – even bulk varieties bought in health food stores – add way too much. Often it's better to make your own granola.

Next add in some fruit. Bananas, apples, pears work – as do many others. Dried fruits are useful, but often studded with HFCS – so use them sparingly.

Want to add nuts? Please do. Almonds and walnuts get first priority.

Next, try different milks. Skim milk can be mixed with soymilk. Plant-based milks – like soy and almond milk – also can mix very well.

The more you put stuff together, the richer and often the sweeter the taste. For people with a sweet tooth – like me – that matters a lot.

Breakfast is also a nice time for coffee or tea. Half of America's antioxidants come from coffee, which seems to have protective effects against diabetes and Parkinsonism among other nasty diseases.

Make your breakfast pretty big – if you can, the biggest meal of the day. If you make breakfast the largest daily meal you may discover a really good way to help control weight.

So write down what you had for Breakfast

_____

_____

Next up – Lunch – the perfect time for nutritional variety –

Drink water – a full glass – before you eat.

Lunch is also a good time for fish – like a small 3-ounce tin of sardines.

Then add your five colors.

Include multiple vegetables – like spinach, kale, celery, carrots, broccoli, green beans, cauliflower.

Fruits – get what's in season – but apples, oranges, and bananas are often available and generally cost less. Lunch can be made more attractive by adding small bits of more expensive fruits like kiwi, berries and apricots. Add colors for beauty – and varied foods that give your body the right information for proper regeneration.

Be careful around starches like bread and pasta. As far as your body is concerned they quickly turn into glucose. Remember how quickly sugar becomes fat – especially when you take in a lot at once.

Add beans – virtually any kind. Pinto beans, lentils, navy beans, black beans, fava beans – there's a very long list to choose from.

Finish the meal with a fruit you love or a few nuts. I like apples to end a meal as they can help clean up your teeth – though flossing after a meal also helps.

Doctors don't talk much about teeth. They should. Teeth are very important to overall health.

So what did you eat for Lunch?

Supper:

This is the time when most people have time to cook.

So think:

A small, varied salad to start the meal.

Cooked vegetables. Stews.

Big simmering pots of lentils and beans – spiced with peppers and chilies.

Small amounts of delicious fish – like salmon. If you can afford the wild variety, cook with the goal of 3-4 ounces per person.

Finish the meal with a fruit, nuts, a nice glass of brewed herbal or green tea (you probably want that decaffeinated – sleep is as necessary to your life as food).

So what did you eat for Supper?

_____

_____

Snacks

If you're diabetic, snacks may be necessary. If you eat five or six meals – regularly and to a regular schedule – snacks may be what you do.

Otherwise – *avoid them.*

Sometimes you can't. So think of a fistful of –

- Wasabi peas
- Almonds
- Walnuts
- Soy nuts

- Cut carrots
- A long stick of celery

Each can be a decent snack.

Overview

If you had –

Breakfast every morning; tried to put different colors on your plate each meal; drank coffee or tea most mornings –

You're doing OK.

If you had –

A large breakfast most mornings, with different cereals and nuts and fruits; controlled snack intake; had at most one alcoholic drink six or less nights a week; ate a salad with different colors on it several days a week –

You're doing well.

If you had –

A multiple-colored breakfast every morning; ate multiple fruit or vegetables or cereals at virtually every meal; tried five colors on your supper plate at least four times a week –

You're doing very well.

If you had –

Two or three different kinds of fruit, or cereal, or vegetables with each meal; put five colors on most of your plates; did not snack –

You're doing really well.

And you'll be doing better still. For health is about synergy – not just what you eat and when, but combining that with how you move – how you rest – and how you socialize.

Put them together and overall function improves further. You'll start to see how in the next chapter – on Exercise. Physical activity changes how you obtain food – and especially what your body does with it.

Want to control weight and feel energetic? Read on.

Because it's a joy to own your body – to do fun things with it – and rebuild it the way you like. Putting food together with physical activity makes it all that much easier.

Chapter 4 – Exercise

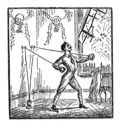

You've been sold a bill of goods.

Does health come out of a pill bottle? No more than exercise magically pours forth from a gym.

Gyms can be grand and gyms can be grim, but gyms are not necessary for great physical activity.

Let's illustrate. **Which of these is "exercise?"**

1. Running the Antarctic marathon (suitably dressed).

2. Escaping from a noisy pub.

3. Cleaning the dishes.

4. Talking at curbside to your elderly neighbor.

5. Fidgeting in front of a movie theater, figuring out which ticket you and your boy/girlfriend want to buy.

The answer is – *all of these*. All are exercise. Exercise is anything that puts your voluntary muscles into action.

Which includes reading the last sentence out loud.

Yes, your tongue and lips are voluntary muscles – with many uses beyond speech.

And fidgeting counts – quite a bit, if the data from Mayo Clinic can be believed. So does standing. Standing all by itself takes 25% more energy than sitting. All these movements represent different forms of exercise.

One thing you really don't want to do is sit very long.

Sitting Can Kill You

If you don't believe me, ask a truck driver. About 86% of American truck drivers are overweight.

Truck drivers and people who sit at work – or for frequent entertainment – are literal sitting ducks.

So are you and I. Sitting – at least while you're awake – is a hazard to your health. Sit long, live less.

The numbers truly are troubling. At leisure, folks who sit more than six hours a day die earlier. The increase in male mortality is 17%; female mortality, 37% (no, life is not fair). And the longer you sit, the quicker you die.

This is even true of regular exercisers. Yes, marathon runners who sit a lot will die earlier than they could or should.

So it's time to grow to enjoy your hunter-gatherer body, built to walk the earth, swim the oceans, and sprint across mountain ridges. **Your body is a walking machine.** It is built to move.

And it likes doing it. A lot.

Talk to professional athletes. Many claim to enjoy their outrageous paychecks, the eye-turning celebrity, the screams of fans when they make the right moves.

But most of them will tell you they what they really love is playing the game. They love the action, the intense excitement, the exaltation from skilled, sudden movement. For many athletes, exercise is much more than a job – it is *pure exhilaration.*

That can be your experience, too.

Benefits and Privileges

There are other benefits to moving rather than sitting, like:

Long life – some estimates are that regular physical activity of many kinds – which you'll learn is not difficult to do – adds six to seven years to life.

Looking good – Our image of health and beauty has changed. It is no longer the voluptuous, small pot-bellied belles of the Renaissance nor the twigged out heroin chic pencil-armed stick figures of a few years ago.

These days movie stars work out.

Beauty has become much closer to classical Greek ideas – trim, muscular, quick limbed. Even if people don't look "athletic," the healthy glow that comes to your skin after a quick hike upstairs makes most folks look more alive and attractive.

So remember, exercise makes you look good – and all voluntary motion constitutes exercise.

Weight control – Only two-thirds of Americans are officially overweight, but even when you aren't, keeping yourself in good shape is usually important for getting into the same wardrobe year after year. Want to lose 30 pounds and really keep it off? Walk an hour a day more than you do now. Exercise intensely and you can burn fat for many hours – after you stop.

Better skin – Walk around – especially if you know how to use the sun rather than be damaged by it – and your skin will be more taut and clear. That gives you a much better shot at looking like those preposterously young kids in skin cream commercials.

Fewer heart attacks

Fewer strokes

Less cancer

Less depression – walking in morning light is probably as or more effective than many drugs for mild to moderate clinical depression.

Fewer colds – plus moving around a bit when you've got one makes the symptoms less unpleasant.

Better bones and fewer fractures

Better muscles and joints – especially for the long haul of long life.

More brown fat – Exercise regularly and you can change white fat to mitochondria-laden brown fat. Brown fat burns off calories far more quickly.

Changing the color of your fat is a bigger trick than changing the color of your eyes – and it can really change how you feel.

Where Can You Go? Exercise Everywhere for Energy and Exhilaration

One of the cool things about exercise is that it involves most every voluntary motion you make – even ones, like fidgeting, that you may not be aware you're doing.

So exercise can include almost everything you do – besides sleeping, that is.

The next cool thing about exercise is that you can do it everywhere – all you need is space to move.

Standing is exercise – as well as an opportunity to relax and concentrate. But lots of us spend our time sitting at desks, on dining room chairs or scrunched atop sofas.

So *don't think conventionally.* You shouldn't – especially if your goal is to remain healthy and not see the extraordinarily expensive insides of a hospital.

Recognize that exercise happens doing the most ordinary things – in slightly less ordinary ways.

I used to think that typing my books and articles required me to sit at a desk. At least I needed a chair.

Wrong. I'm writing this standing in front of my bright, inexpensive computer monitor perched on a lovely red glass and steel adjustable desk. I can quickly convert it into an ordinary sitting desk – whenever I like.

Though I don't want it to become a conventional desk. When I type standing I feel more alert. I can pace a little while I tickle the keys, twist or turn my body at will; practice yoga standing poses; even dance to music inside my head or popping from my laptop.

Sitting, I rarely feel so free. When I stand and write I do feel free – free to move, to riff, to stretch and sway.

I'm also exercising.

Where You Spend Your Day

Though Americans would prefer a 26- or at least a 25-hour day, including at least an extra hour for the rest their body needs to regenerate but which they generally neglect to obtain (please see the next chapter), 24 hours is still a lot of time. What kinds and amount of movement maximizes lifespan?

Somewhere between 60-90 minutes of physical activity. Which means about 6% of your waking hours.

For a body that's built to be a walking machine, that's a piddling amount.

Especially because you can get those minutes almost everywhere you go.

So where do you spend your day?

Chained to a desk at work? Chained to a desk at school?

Or are you spending oodles of hours sitting in front of a TV set or computer monitor? If you do, you've got company – Americans have their TV sets on for more than eight hours a day.

Or perhaps you're stuck in a car, commuting to work or taking the kids to school?

Perhaps you're a teenager doing your requisite two to three hours of texting each day? Or an involuntary housewife – right now you simply can't find a job – sitting and drinking coffee at the dining room table?

So tote up the minutes you spend sitting at

Work	____
School	____
In the Car	____
Watching TV	____
Surfing or working the Net	____
Ensconced in your chair eating	____

Pretty large number? Perhaps most of your daytime day?

Don't despair. You're now going to learn how to turn those activities into healthy, simple, easy-to-do exercise.

Turning Your Home Into Your Private Gym

Every step you take counts. And you can take a lot of steps at home.

Want to improve mood, alertness? Decrease your risk of depression and reset the internal clocks that time your life?

When you wake in the morning, get on some old clothes and walk outside.

Too cold or too dark out there? Move inside the house.

Yes, you can walk back and forth in the living room or around the other rooms. You can walk up and down an apartment building or your home's stairs. But to get always accessible, more intense exercise, it's often easier to use some type of athletic equipment. Exercycles, treadmills, and elliptical machines are expensive. They get a lot less expensive after Christmas – especially secondhand. You'll be surprised what's available for $100-$200 when a machine is no longer new – and sometimes all the use it got was being taken out of the box and positioned as a clothes hanger.

If you do get an exercise machine, find one you can read on. That helps many work and move at the same time. Pedaling or walking 20 or 30 minutes will also grow you new brain cells – in memory areas – during the night (one thing sleep is for).

Moving twenty to thirty minutes a day increases your brain's information storage and helps prevent stroke, heart attack, and cancer simultaneously. Not bad.

And if you think you're too tired to move – exercise will usually pep you up. Physical effort can overcome mental fatigue. Unless done to extremes, exercise literally helps shape the body's necessary regeneration – in healthy ways.

Exercise machines have the advantage of negating bad weather as an obstacle to even the most intense physical activity. It can be snowing or storming outside, but you can choose the type of activity you want.

If you can't afford or don't like any athletic equipment, get a step. You can buy a plastic step – which automatically becomes a stepper – for less than $10. Any time you can stand you can also step. Then you just step on your stepper with your right foot – and step off. Next, step on and off with your left.

Repeat.

If that demands too much attention from whatever else you're doing, just work one foot at a time. If you can't afford a stepper, an old, thick book you no longer care to read will suffice (this book is too small for that purpose – even if it's packed with other kinds of energy).

Eating

Exercise while you're eating? Don't even think of it – in Japan. Walk and eat at the same time and little kids will point their fingers at you, amazed at such tasteless, uncivilized behavior.

Other places it's a different story.

We've been taught to sit down to our meals. We've also been taught to sit "long enough for digestion."

Good advice – when you don't get enough food to eat. There are at least six million households in the U.S. where people go to bed hungry several times each week.

But for most of us eating and then sitting – like a stone – is precisely the wrong advice.

People have and will assume almost any position while eating.

And eating standing up – better, standing after you've eaten – can prevent gastroesophageal reflux disease (GERD) by as much as 50%.

Certainly most of us cook standing up. And though at first it may seem unsociable, standing up during mealtimes can provide exercise – even if it's just to get the next course.

It's even better to become active following the meal. And better yet to socially stroll – with family or friends.

The advantages of moving after meals are almost too long a list. If you move around, particularly walking following a meal, you:

• Increase blood flow to the arms and legs – which results in less blood flow to the gut –

Which Means

• Lower glucose peaks in your blood

• Lower insulin and insulin growth factor peaks

• Less fat added to your abdomen. And since visceral fat is an endocrine gland, which tends to make you bigger, moving after meals is one of the most effective weight control strategies available to you, which

• Also helps prevent GERD

• Helps grow more brain cells

- Converts white fat cells to faster burning brown fat cells
- Improves mood – especially if you move in sunlight

Television

Want to get heart disease? Sit down in front of the TV every day for a few hours – especially after a long day at work.

You might be able to double your chance of coronary artery disease – just by becoming a perfectly ordinary couch potato.

Yet no one has decreed you must sit in a chair or lounge on a sofa to watch TV.

When you watch, you can stand.

People don't think they can exercise when they watch TV. That only happens in gyms, right?

No. Here are some activities you can try while watching the tube or computer monitor:

• Want to improve balance? Stand on one foot for five seconds. Then stand on the other. Later, with practice, do it for 10 seconds or longer on each foot.

• You can stand and watch while moving back and forth on a stepper.

• You can watch while "sitting" on an exercycle, or moving on a treadmill or elliptical machine.

• You can do yoga positions – particularly standing yoga positions – as you watch.

• You can lift small weights - one, two, or if you're so minded, five or 10 pounds – side to side or curling at your shoulders – while you watch.

Don't want to stand while watching your favorite soap opera? *What are commercials for – if not opportunities to move around?*

If standing, standing and stepping, or running back and forth to the kitchen for a nice snack of fennel or celery is insufficiently energizing, you can do squats. Squats can be done with great intensity.

And the amazing thing about intense exercise is that it provokes fat burning – long after you've stopped moving. So if you feel you've sat too long, go and try squats for one to two minutes.

In those 120 seconds you may miss some stunning pharmaceutical ads showing pretty people in gorgeous Hawaiian scenery, or some political sound bites on why candidate X is much, much nastier than all the creatures sucked out of the Black Lagoon.

But you'll be moving.

Computers

Surfing the Net? Standing beats sitting. Stepping beats standing.

Dancing beats them all.

Humans love music. We love music in part because we are fundamentally rhythmic. Our biology is intensely rhythmic.

Time rules life. Listening to music while you're on the Net may improve your concentration.

But bopping a little while you type can help you stay slim; look good; improve your mood; and keep you moving more.

Endurance goes up when people exercise and listen to music – especially when doing intense exercise. Set the rhythm speed to 120-135 beats a minute – and watch yourself go.

Cars

Most car manufacturers want to turn your vehicle into a roaming "technology center." By barking one or two syllables you can change the TV channels or discover the highway exit to the closest pizza joint.

Resist the temptation to become an instant cyborg.

Car companies will make a lot of money from such technology "add-ons" but they're often taking you away from healthy activities.

I deliberately bought mechanical windows for my car. I need the exercise more than my car engine.

That way the *electricity comes from inside me.*

Mechanical windows are now as common as vacuum tubes (can't remember them?), but since all muscle movements are exercise, use them when you can.

Seatbelts are necessary to your health and safety – put them on first. But sadly, cars don't give you many opportunities to move around. Look at truck drivers – and their often horrible health.

If you like to dance, put dance music on the radio and rhythmically move in your seat. If that feels strange, sing. Even if you're the worst karaoke singer in the Western hemisphere, when the windows are rolled up few people will know – or be bothered.

And singing can improve mood; some folks even use it to decrease depression.

Music – especially when internally generated – gives you something fun to do when you're commuting in a car.

Texting and Cell Phones

Do not text and drive. Period. Texting and driving can put you and several others into the hospital, a place you do not want to stay in even if you could pay for it. And sometimes the outcome is worse – you never make it to the hospital at all.

Walking while texting, though it violates the brain's "you can only do one thing at a time" rule, is a combined activity some of us can manage. Of course, you need to be moving in a place where you won't bump into something dangerous. Otherwise you risk becoming sudden, inadvertent road kill.

So it's generally better to talk on the phone, rather than text, while on the move. This can be accomplished at home, at the mall, on the street, in gardens, forests, woods, beaches, open plazas, office buildings, postal branches and Department of Motor Vehicle Offices – though not in the last spot if you're waiting in line.

Lyndon Johnson said of future President Gerry Ford, "That man can't walk and chew bubble gum at the same time."

Gerry Ford could. And most all of us can walk and talk into a cell phone at the same time.

Connecting with the people we love, like, or merely need to connect with. And simultaneously moving, which helps our hearts;

our brain arteries; our brains; our muscles; our waistlines – all as we socially connect.

As you'll learn later, social connection can be *really regenerative* – and healthy.

Self-Transport

It's a simple principle – you need exercise more than your car; your motorcycle; your scooter; your RV; SUV; golf cart; or your ATV.

Self-transport – generally walking or biking – can do more than make you look good, feel good, control your waistline, and prevent the most common fatal and chronic diseases known to man.

It's also good for the planet.

Sure, walking or biking takes energy. Energy requires food. Some commentators will even offer you bizarre, false statistical arguments that it's environmentally better to drive than for you to get to where you want entirely under your own steam.

Don't believe such nonsense. New Yorkers live about two-and-a-half years longer than other Americans.

Obviously that's because New York is such a stress-free, calm, relaxed, happy, euphoria-inducing town, right?

A more likely reason is that getting almost anywhere in New York involves moving your own carcass part of the way.

Owning a car in New York is expensive; parking is expensive; parking your car away from home can be ruinously expensive.

So New Yorkers use buses, and trains, often taxis.

And when you take the subway, you generally need to go up and down stairs. And to get to and from buses you must walk – and often stand as you wait for them.

So a little movement goes a long way – for your health – and the health of the place you live.

Self-transport will add very little carbon dioxide to the atmosphere. It can make you happy, quick, sometimes exhilarated.

As well as a little proud you're getting somewhere on your own two feet.

You don't have to move fast. Australian researchers argue that, at least among the old, three miles an hour separates the quick and the dead.

If you're young, you can go faster.

Exercise at Work

Think of your office building as a massive workout space.

There should be a stairs somewhere – or two or three. Conference rooms. Long corridors.

Which means plenty of space in which to move.

Stairs are particularly efficient exercise arenas. You can move up and down; slowly or rapidly; one or two steps at a time (be careful of aging joints when choosing the last option).

Chained to a desk? You can talk *and* walk while on the phone. And sometimes you need to recognize the requirements of nature. Many of us who are middle aged can find a bathroom sufficiently far away that we may get a sizable percentage of our daily exercise performed very readily.

You can walk to a bathroom, of course; but you can also skip, or jog, or even race a bit. Too embarrassed to skip down a corridor? Find a stairwell landing that is anonymous and private, and you should be able to move about whatever way you like.

And despite some older corporate practices, it really pays to talk to people face to face. Use that argument to get your body moving when outside the building, but also to meet everyone inside your office. You never know what they might tell you about the boss, impending layoffs, or just where the best parties are.

Working in a small office? Get to know your neighbors. *Stroll on by and say hi.* You might discover all kinds of useful things about your landlord, parking spaces, or where the healthiest restaurants are.

And when you do have time for lunch, try to find a place you can walk to – and walk back from. Bring along a work colleague – or two or three. Go visit a friend or acquaintance. You can also bring a bag lunch and picnic in a park – if the weather is agreeable – or find an indoor office plaza with seating if it's not.

To exercise and simultaneously relax, find yourself a yoga mat. Try doing simple yoga positions at your job, before and after work. All you need is a three by six-foot space. If your boss recognizes what the increased relaxation and concentration does for your productivity, you may also get to do yoga during work. A few minutes of yoga and stretching every two to three hours can make a big difference in your effectiveness, state of mind, balance and flexibility.

Once you begin to think about it, you can find places to move almost anywhere.

Though some places are tough.

Airplanes

Unless you're willing to pay a lot for legroom, airplanes are unfriendly to exercise.

You just have to make them so.

With the exception of really wanting to sleep for a while, try to get an aisle seat. According to microbiologists, aisle seats may make you prone to meeting more bacteria, viruses and fungi from other passengers. That's probably a small price to pay. Aisle seats make it a lot easier to move when on a plane.

To prevent clots, try to get up from your seat every one to two hours. Walk to the further bathroom or galley – even if you have need of neither.

Generally you can do stretching at the sides of airplane galleys, or next to your plane's rear emergency exit doors. If the bathroom is vacant, you can do knee bends and different kinds of squats inside that very small space.

Yoga moves generally require a three by six foot space – the edges of the galley at the rear of a plane will usually suffice.

While in your seat, you can bring small weights – or just use books, laptops, or tablets as your exercise weights. When you can, pump your legs.

Blood clots acquired on planes are more common than people know, though few turn out to be truly dangerous. *When in doubt, move whatever muscles you can* – and get on friendly relations with your seatmates – especially during a long flight. Both can help calm the mind and pass the time.

If You Simply Will Not Exercise, Get a Dog

Pets are great.

An internist cousin says he knows who amongst his elderly patients will live longer.

They have dogs.

Cats can be wonderful, too. Owning a pet lowers blood pressure; decreases stress; often increases your social support.

But many people seem congenitally incapable of moving.

Dogs make you walk.

Not only must you walk a dog (unless you have a large yard – which is cheating) but also you must walk with your dog more than once a day.

By walking a dog you will –

- Help clean up your arteries
- Grow new brain cells
- Decrease your risk of Alzheimer's disease
- Decrease your risk of death
- Get mood enhancing sunshine (at least sometimes)
- Reset and synchronize body clocks

And there's more:

1. Cats, dogs and other pets can provide love – and then some. It now appears from genetic studies that primates – apes, including humans – have rather similar genes controlling social structures. They're old. Some of these genes may go back 50 million years.

We are social animals.

We apply these social structures to more than just people – we apply them to the animals in our lives.

Dogs have been co-evolving with us for at least 17,000 years. As we have bred them to become more dependent, they have learned a lot about us – and know more things than we can know.

That's because dogs and cats have a very developed smell brain – they navigate much of life with their nose.

They may smell pheromones (airborne hormones) that we can't. They can tell by smell, vision and gesture when we're distressed – often before we do. And they often come around to try and make us feel better.

2. With their smell brains, short attention spans, and wandering ways, dogs meet other dogs – whom we ourselves meet.

We also get to meet their owners.

Many a love match has come to people through their dogs – and many a social connection important to their lives.

3. Dogs and cats can be great for kids – providing affection and a chance for them to exercise and learn responsibility – and develop regular habits.

So pets promote love, social connection, and social rest – relieving stress, lowering blood pressure, and often making us much happier.

Figure on $20-$30 bucks a month on food for dogs and cats, especially the high-end stuff. Vet visits and vaccines will add at least $100 a year. With age and any trouble, figure on $400-$500 a year in vet bills.

Getting a pet may be one of the best investments you ever make.

Wear a Hat

Who gets skin cancer? Most people who live long – and quite a few others. Most skin cancers will appear on the face, ears and neck.

You can prevent a lot of them by wearing a hat whenever you're outside – and prevent a lot of skin damage, too.

Most people never take this simple, easy precaution. Many men consider wearing hats, except for baseball caps, rather odd. Yet any movie buff can tell you **not** wearing a hat was a pretty gauche move throughout much of the 20th century.

Women don't like hats for several reasons – with hairstyles number one. Hats are considered *hairdo killers*.

Nonsense.

Look at hats and their historical fashion and practical importance. Women have worn hats everywhere and in every period. Hats have been accessorized at least as much as shoes. Magnificent hats have graced aristocratic and middle class households for thousands of years.

If you like shoes, you may come to love hats. They can provide you a different look every day of the year.

And hairstyles can be accommodated to them – quickly.

Besides, melanomas are more than deadly – they can also be disfiguring, as are basal and squamous cell skin cancers. Greater sun exposure also leads to darkened, coarsened, even leathery skin – especially for those of us who live in the South. Wide brimmed hats can really decrease that risk.

Yes, you do want light on your eyes – where it can improve mood and reset clocks, as well as spark up your natural killer cells to fight off some rather unpleasant viruses (though high levels of direct sunlight may help form cataracts). You just don't need that much light elsewhere on your skin – though bits of sunlight will help you make vitamin D.

Hats can be stylish, fun, provide you with better looking skin, and prevent cancer.

They're a good deal.

Summary

Exercise is any use of voluntary muscle. It includes fidgeting and walking, strolling and standing. With very few exceptions, the more you get, the better.

Mice who exercise immediately increase their number of cellular recyclers, called autophagosomes. That directly aids their regeneration.

And just as exercise includes virtually all your motions, virtually any environment can be used to exercise. You can even exercise in cars and on planes - or watching the NFL.

We're walking machines. **Use your body the way it's built and it will thank you.**

You'll also look better – and regenerate better. Every time you move a muscle you influence its future remaking – usually in a positive way. Exercise lets you change your inner tissues – and your shape. You give your body new information on how to reorganize and re-form itself – especially your brain. Move enough and you grow new brain cells – probably one of the many reasons physical activity is so helpful in blocking and treating depression. Even people with chronic illnesses can usually do some form of physical activity. Most of these actions aid health.

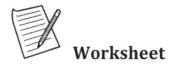 **Worksheet**

If you recognize that exercise is any use of voluntary muscle you've come a long way.

Standing is exercise.

Walking is exercise.

Talking in the hallway is exercise.

Moving to the bathroom is exercise.

Here are a few suggestions for your day:

Morning

Before breakfast – try a few stretches – then put on some old clothes and walk.

Aim for 10-15 minutes of walking, housework, or yard work – if you can. Try walking or biking to a specific destination – like a wood, park, or friends' house. Or doing a specific project – like clearing leaves from the driveway. Five minutes of activity can be quite useful. Get outside when possible.

Can't get outside? Do at least 10 minutes on a

- Stepper (you can watch the morning news)
- Exercycle
- Elliptical
- Treadmill – or exercise machine of your choice

After breakfast

Walk if you can – outdoor sunlight is usually more effective than indoor sunlight (wear a hat outside – unless it's dark). Try to get in at least five minutes of some physically active activity. You can clear up clutter, tidy up the kitchen. Keep standing if possible to limit GERD.

If you can walk 10-15 minutes, you'll be doing your waistline a favor – and decreasing your risk of heart disease.

If possible, walk or bicycle to work. Too far? Find an intermediate spot to park your car – or use public transport.

Self-transport is better for you and your community.

Write down **your exercise before and after breakfast**

_____

_____

At Work

Get out of your seat whenever possible. Stand at least every hour. Try for at least a minute each hour where you're not sitting.

Stand or walk around if you're talking on the telephone – and you don't need to write or watch a monitor.

Go for a two to three minute walk at least once before lunch – if it's difficult to do anything else, go to the bathroom furthest away.

Take the stairs to any meeting. Can't go the whole way? Do as many flights as you can to make yourself more alert.

When possible, do yoga postures for 30-60 seconds once before lunch.

Your exercise at work

_____

_____

Lunch

Use self-transport. Walk or bike to a restaurant, or park, or picnic spot. Aim for 10 minutes each way.

Remember – a 20-minute walk can grow you new brain cells. The way the world is going, you'll need them.

Your exercise at lunch

_____

_____

Afternoon

If you have headphones or accessible music – and nobody is watching – try to dance for at least a minute – even if it's at your desk (and your boss and co-workers can't see you – or don't mind).

Stand at least once an hour.

Walk over to a work colleague for a minute or two – and talk. Ask them how they are – and mean it. It's generally better to talk face to face than by telephone.

Get in at least one two-to-three minute walk to a bathroom or stairwell.

At the end of the day, stand up and think about what you've accomplished that day – and what you want to accomplish the next day – for at least one minute.

When possible, go home by self-transport – walking or biking.

Your afternoon exercise

_____

_____

Evening

After the evening meal, stroll with family or friends. It's best done outside – and as socially as you can. Aim for 10 to 15 minutes – at the least.

If watching TV, stand for a while. Use a stepper for at least five minutes of a program. Treadmills or elliptical machines are even better – generally the longer they're used, the more beneficial the effect.

Do some standing yoga poses when watching TV or looking at the Net.

Invite a friend over. If the weather is good, walk around the neighborhood.

Your evening exercise

_____

_____

When you can

It's certainly fun to swim. Getting into a heated pool two to three times a week can do wonders for joints and flexibility.

If you can –

Walk five or 10 minutes every morning; walk back and forth to lunch; stand at different intervals during the day –

You're doing OK.

If you can –

Walk ten or fifteen minutes after at least two meals each day; stand or walk around your office or workplace every hour; and stroll sometimes with a friend –

You're doing well.

If you can –

Walk or move at least 45 minutes a day; stand or walk every hour on the job; do a few minutes of yoga every day –

You're doing very well.

If you can –

Walk to work or friends' houses; move at least an hour a day; walk with your friends or family after the evening meal; view your workplace and your home as good places to keep moving –

You're doing really well.

Exercise remakes your body and mind. It can literally change your tissues – as it does shifting white fat to brown. It grows brain cells, strengthens muscles, decreases anxiety – and for many provides some of the peak physical and social experiences of their lives.

It regenerates you. And much of it costs not a penny.

But just like morning needs night, activity needs rest. Rest is also required to rebuild and regenerate your body.

It's also fun – as you'll soon see.

Chapter 5 - Exciting Rest

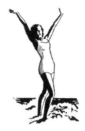

What do fast food companies, cosmetics dealers, energy drink manufacturers, cookie confectioners, and oil behemoths have in common?

At least two things: they make or use oil and gas – and employ petrochemicals in their products.

And all of them can potentially make boatloads of money keeping you awake.

Fast food companies can hugely increase their profits because sleeping poorly makes people weigh more, which causes them to buy more food; poor sleep makes you absolutely crave sugary and fatty foods, the stuff they specialize in. Sleeping less causes you to make more bad decisions and take riskier risks, making it easier to sell products to exhausted insomniacs.

Cosmetics sellers do well too; sleeplessness makes people look lousy. One quick and supposedly easy way to look better is to buy more – and more expensive – cosmetics.

Energy drink manufacturers get an especially special "no way we can lose" business deal. Keeping folks up at night makes it easier to sell energy drinks, which make people even more sleepless – which means they need *yet more* energy drinks. The added weight and frequent fatigue that accompanies poor sleep also makes it easier to sell "energy" in a can.

Cookie makers really have come to relish a heavier population that wants more sugary foods. TV production chiefs want you up at night so they can sell you more advertising. They need your eyeballs open! **Remember – poor sleep also leads to weight gain.** People who weigh more have more inflammatory markers in their blood – and sleep even less. That makes them perfect marks for infomercials blasting in the middle of the night. And it's far simpler to sell Ginsu knives (It Slices! It Dices!) and hair growth gels to sleepless people because they make less rational decisions, as military research has painfully revealed.

Oil companies make billions each year selling the petrochemicals put into food, cosmetics, televisions and the like. But they really like selling oil and gas. And a weightier population takes more energy – to make, transport, and cook the added food they eat. You then have to move, heat and cool those millions of expanded bodies. By some estimates, add a pound to the U.S. population and you may add a couple of billion dollars in energy costs – every year.

So there are lots of people who can and will make money on keeping you sleepless. That's not to mention sleeping pill manufacturers and the concocters of the 390 "relaxation drinks" that supposedly help you slumber.

Don't want to gain weight, look worse, feel and perform worse *and* become financially poorer? *Thwart 'em all: it's time to learn to rest naturally.*

And once you can do that you'll also have a much better shot at less heart disease; fewer strokes; fewer colds; fewer severe infections; less depression. And those are just the side benefits of re-learning how to rest.

Why re-learn? Because rest used to be as easy and unthinking as breathing. It's time to reclaim control, take charge over your body – and really enjoy yourself.

Rest has two major components – active and passive. The form you probably know best is the passive rest we call sleep.

Sleep deprive animals and they die. **You really do need sleep like food.** The trick is getting the right amount and the right kind of rest to regenerate yourself – and to make the process fun. Rest should provide at least as many pleasures as dining – and deeper ones.

So let's answer some of the most common FAQs:

1. How much sleep do I need?

Probably more than you get. Teenagers and early twenty-somethings probably need nine to nine-and-a-half hours on average to fully learn, control weight and be completely functional; seventy-somethings might make out well getting something between seven and eight hours. But those are just population averages. One of my friends, now 71, needs three hours a night, the same as his 97-year-old mother and 75-year-old brother. My friend and his brother are both very high functioning physicians – who work fulltime.

2. How do I figure out how much sleep I personally need?

Remember the last time you took a real vacation? One where you *really felt rested?*

Don't include the first four or five days – in these economic times many use the first part of vacations to overcome chronic sleep deprivation. When you're finally doing stuff you really like and can fully control your time, you'll get a pretty good idea of how many hours of sleep your body needs.

Still can't figure it out? Try sleeping eight full hours for a week and see if you feel fully rested when you wake up. Then you can figure if your need is more than that – or less.

3. If I can't get enough sleep at night, can I make up for the sleep loss by sleeping during the day?

Yes – to a point. Just as people "pig out" during the holidays, they "sleep out" on the weekends, sleeping more hours during the mornings or, better, taking naps. Sadly, there's a price for that – blowing out your biological clocks. People go to bed later on Friday and Saturday nights, and get up later. Then Monday morning arrives – the peak time of death in the U.S., with heart attack rates increasing as much as five times.

Trust me – regular schedules can help keep you healthy.

4. What are the best kinds of naps?

Short ones. Long naps bring out sleep inertia – that dead, leaden feeling – kind of like a hangover – that comes with naps lasting long enough to reach deeper phases of sleep. Fifteen or 20-minute naps help many revive. Folks who routinely get more than an hour's nap *may* disrupt their body clocks and lessen night-time sleep, which can knock the whole process out of whack (it's a different story for shift workers).

To keep naps short, use a kitchen timer or your cell phone as timing device.

5. What's the simplest advice for getting good sleep?

Go to bed and get up at the same times seven nights a week. We did not evolve with weekends. In recent laboratory experiments that mimic pre-industrial days people went to bed a bit after sunset, woke up at night to think about dreams, got up at dawn and napped during the day. Many had very pleasant spiritual experiences. Our present day version of sleep – sometimes called the American "lie down and die" model – has little to do with how we would naturally sleep.

As the Romans said, times rules life. To make sleep efficient set things up so body clocks are regular. Your internal body clocks are a bit like the timer on a mechanical engine – they're just a heckuva lot more important. When clocks are disrupted, many normal functions may go haywire. You might ask shift workers you know – on average they gain more weight, have more heart and GI disease, and perhaps more cancers.

Get your body clocks aligned and you'll feel and look better – and you'll probably perform more productively.

6. What kind of bed environment helps me sleep?

For most folks think of *three Cs – cool, calm, comfortable.* People can and do sleep in hundreds of positions, with extremely varied mattresses, cushions, and sleep paraphernalia. Yet most of us like cool, dark sleeping spaces. Cheap eye masks, which cover the eyes, can be real useful light blockers, whether it's your home, a train, a plane, a bus, or a hotel room. We can easily sense very small amounts of light with our eyes closed.

7. What happens if I can't sleep well most nights?

Join a very, very big club. Maybe a third of the population has lots of trouble sleeping. Ordinary reasons vary from weighing too much and breathing poorly to drinking too much caffeine too late. Others worry about sleep, think a lot about sleep, and fret about sleep – which provokes many to *not sleep.*

Hundreds of medical conditions muck up sleep – especially anything involving pain. **Lots of medications reduce sleep**. That includes many sleeping pills, which can produce their own forms of dependence – along with far from normal sleep.

Yet for most of us sleep functions pretty well if:

• We give it enough time (see section 2 above).

• We move around during the day – even minimally. The fitter you are, the better you sleep.

• Your bed environment is protected and pleasing.

• You stop turning sleep into a job and make it a pleasure. *Turn sleep into work – or a work project – and it doesn't happen.*

8. How can I make sleep fun?

If you could remember all the different forms of consciousness you get during a single night's sleep, you might imagine you led several different interesting lives.

Part of sleep's importance is that it rewires much of your brain and body. *You learn during sleep.* You remake memories, along with your joints, muscles, and skin. Skin really grows fast at night.

To have fun with sleep it's a good idea to focus on what's slightly more than a fifth of normal sleep – complex dream sleep, also called REM sleep.

Can't remember your dreams? OK – set your alarm about fifteen minutes earlier than usual. Have pen, pencil and paper nearby. You can also type on your cellphone or tablet, of course – but please keep them off during the night. Night-time texting, emailing, twittering and cellphone conversations can keep you *up most nights – and sleepy all day.*

To make dreaming fun, set your alarm a little earlier than usual. Normally we're deep inside a big, long REM period just before we wake. Wake just a little before that REM period ends and you should be able to remember your dreams. It also helps to immediately write them down.

And before you sleep you can pre-dream – throughout the day. Pre-dreaming means visualizing dreams you'd like to have at night. You can fly to Paris or the moon, visit fantastic countries, or create heroic adventures set in any place, time, or history. Pre-dreaming can also help you achieve your real dreams – at no financial cost.

9. OK, but I'm still waking and staying up in the middle of the night – what do I do when I want to get back to sleep?

Several things including:

1. **Don't look at the clock.** Clockwatching conditions you to wake up at that time each and every night. Instead turn the clock face away or cover it 2. If you wake and are not back to sleep in five to 10 minutes, get out of bed. Beds should be for sleep and sex. Lying in bed waiting for sleep unfortunately can prolong sleeplessness. 3. Next, move from your bed to a place where you can read or listen to music.

What music? There are playlists all over the Net, including a few of my favorites – like the wondrous Hildegard of Bingen.

But reading can really help you sleep.

You just have to choose the right book.

Nothing thrilling, of course. If you're a great mystery fan, don't read mysteries. You want to read something that will really help you fall asleep, like:

• Something you should have read in high school but didn't.

• Art History – pretty pictures combined with text can calm even the chronically over aroused mind.

• Travel books – get some tips for pre-dreaming and place yourself far away from present worries.

• Poetry – *read Longfellow's "Song of Hiawatha" recently? This is your chance.* Rhythmic poetry is often a great way to sleep – unless you get too engaged by what you're reading. Hiawatha is based on the poetic meter of the great Finnish epic, the "Kalevala" – so different from normal English usage that it becomes a fabulous sleep aid (18th century poetry is no piker in this department, either).

• History – Serbian history is not everyone's favorite "glass of tea," but you have to hand it to a country where only one king died a natural death. There are thousands of civilizations out there to read and think about – which can aid slumber throughout the night.

- Memoirs – I keep Harry Truman's on my night table. Biographies and autobiographies often fit the sleep-enhancing bill.

- Books about music and mathematics – Gauss was great, and so was Heinrich Schutz. Yet both can become helpful subjects to read about when you can't sleep.

- Many patients, to help them return to sleep, have used books by Matthew Edlund – like "**The Power of Rest's**" section on sleep. Others tell me that "**The Body Clock Advantage**" is occasionally a helpful sleep aid, and that "**Psychological Time and Mental Illness**" possesses several passages that aid slumber.

10. I'm still not sleeping. What else can I do to really help sleep?

Rest before sleep.

Most of us can easily become hyper aroused. Our physical and mental states frequently are neither calm nor collected. *It's really hard to slumber when you can't turn off your brain.*

So learn to turn off lots of things before you sleep. Start with your preferred electronic devices.

Next, take a half hour to an hour before your preferred bedtime and make it your own, special rest time.

During this rest time you can:

- Pre-dream.

- Turn down the bed.

- Floss and brush your teeth.

- Pick out your clothes for the next day.

- Take off your cosmetics.

- Turn down the lights (Lights don't just keep you up – they reset the internal clocks that time your life).

- Read books like those above, listen to music – or do both.

Engage a few of these actions and you've created your own private sleep ritual – a conditioning set of behaviors that will help you get proper sleep.

And you can always add a just before bedtime hot bath. Make sure the water is hot enough – and you soak long enough – to sweat.

Sweating means your body core temperature goes up – and then swiftly lurches down. As studies by Janet Mullington and others show, swift nighttime cooling appears to make us wake less often; increases deep sleep, when we preferentially secrete growth hormone, which may help keep us looking young; and increases REM sleep.

Then when you get up in the morning, put on some old clothes and go (outside if possible) for a morning walk. Morning walks reset body clocks; increase alertness; improve immune function; and help prevent depression.

Morning walks also help you sleep better.

Sleep remakes you. You get a new body and brain when you wake up – literal regeneration. That's not just fun, it's good for your health and spirit.

And when you wake you can start to enjoy rest beyond sleep – active rest.

Active Rest

Rest can be active and exciting – once you know how to do it. Active rest lets you direct how you remake and renew your body – or gets you calm and relaxed when you're ready to jump out the window.

I have a whole book out on active rest – **"The Power of Rest"**. It describes dozens of different active rest techniques and how to do them – reliably – in less than a minute. If you can't afford the book, it's available in most libraries. But here are three quick active rest techniques most folks can do anywhere and any time – as long as you're awake and alert. They provide a *very small* taste of what's available for three different kinds of active rest – physical rest, where you pay attention to your body; mental rest, where you focus on something outside your body; and spiritual rest, where you connect with something larger than yourself. The fourth kind of rest, social rest, is examined in the next chapter.

1. **Physical Rest** – Paradoxical Relaxation

You might have thought PR meant public relations.

PR was devised by Edmund Jacobson, a psychologist and medical physician who became deeply disillusioned with both disciplines. Jacobson trained himself to become relaxed. He became so calm people coming into his presence felt really nervous.

That's real relaxation.

His secret – achieving relaxation without aiming for it – the technique of *paradoxical relaxation.*

Here's a quick way to try it:

Focus on the muscles in your head. Find one that's a little tenser than the one next to it. This muscle can be very small – the tiny, fast moving muscles on the tips of your lips can do nicely – or the often tight muscles of your cheek or jaw.

Now, focus on just this one muscle. Next, close your eyes. As you focus on that muscle, don't relax it, don't tense it – just *feel* it. Visualize it. Feel where the tension starts, peaks, and lessens.

Sense that muscle. Feel it. Know it. Focus on nothing else for 15 seconds.

Now open your eyes.

Feel any relaxation in that muscle?

What about the rest of the body?

The paradox of paradoxical relaxation is that the muscle you've paid attention to may not relax at all – *but the rest of the body probably will.* Withdraw attention from all but one spot and most of your body starts to calm down.

And provides you a quick way to both relaxation and relaxed concentration.

People who use PR practice it by going up and down the body, individual muscle by individual muscle, one at a time. Focusing on one muscle, they get to relax all the others. You can just do five to 20 seconds on one individual muscle – and go to the next.

I certainly would not do PR while in conversation or driving heavy machinery. But you can do it in a surprising number of places – anytime you want. With practice it gets quicker and better – and you do it easily with your eyes open.

You can also use PR to fall asleep.

2. **Mental Rest** - Quick Visualization

I want you to focus on a tree.

Not any tree. It can be the most beautiful tree you remember, a giant chestnut in your grandfather's yard. It can be one you planted in your yard and saw grow to maturity.

It can be the maple or jack pine you view every morning from your bedroom window.

First, see that tree. Notice its trunk, branches, leaves. Find an individual leaf and witness its intricate line of veins – curling and flowing like the circulatory system that keeps you alive.

Now *feel* that tree. Feel the branches sway in a light breeze. Sense the rhythm of its trunk as it moves gradually back and forth, slowly dancing in the air.

Still not relaxed? Imagine your body as the tree. Take your trunk as its trunk, your arms and legs as its branches, your fingers and toes as its leaves. Recognize what it's like to stand powerful and strong, appreciating the changing air while feeling nourished by the sun. Sense the sun on every surface and pore – and the growth it provokes.

After a minute – or less – return back to your own body. Notice how different it feels.

Enjoy the difference.

3. **Spiritual Rest** – Moving in Space

There are many things and places much bigger than we are. Connecting with many of them can provide you a sense of the spiritual – of something greater than oneself – during the most unlikely times, and in the most unusual places.

Please sit down comfortably in a chair.

Notice the room you're in. Inventory in your mind all the different objects – chairs and desks, bookshelves and books, clothing, pictures and rugs. Look at every one of them for the briefest moment – leaving a trace of each in your memory.

Now imagine the neighborhood where you sit. Chances are there are a lot of people around – whether it's a village, town, or city.

Imagine walking – at a calm and deliberate pace – the length and breadth of it.

Where you sit is also part of a larger unit – a state or province. You've got the best walking shoes available in the world, and you decide you will walk its full breadth – at a pace you enjoy.

How long will it take you? Which roads or paths will you choose?

Now imagine you are walking the entire length of the U.S. The United States is 3,000 miles – 5,000 kilometers – long.

Consider what you'll see covering the whole breadth of America. The people you'll meet, the sights, scenes, smells, sounds.

Now do something impossible. Imagine you can – and will – walk to the moon.

You move fairly quickly – four miles an hour. Within a day you've escaped Earth's tiny atmospheric envelope. You've reached space.

It will take you another 2,480 days of non-stop walking to touch the moon's surface.

When you reach it, you'll see the small lunar landers and exploration vehicles people have left there. They are quiet and alone – almost unimaginably remote.

Yet you still will have gotten close to nowhere within our tiny solar system.

And you have not yet started to examine the giant universe of information that lies in the infinite number of spaces smaller than the room where you sit.

For information rules the world – and as physicists will tell you, the entire universe. All that we do, see, say and think is a form of information. And intelligence is the purposeful use of that information.

If you can imagine moving from your seat to the moon, then the intelligence needed to remake your body and health is child's play. A little will and consistent effort, one small bit at a time, is all that's required – **and you will be regenerating yourself following your own direction.**

Best of all, you don't have to do it alone. Humans are profoundly social animals. There are many others who can help you along the way – as you'll learn in the next chapter.

For regeneration is not just physical, mental, and spiritual – it's social. Your friends, family, and colleagues can help you in many ways – including remaking your body and brain in ways you really like.

Summary

Rest, like food, is necessary for life and the full enjoyment of its pleasures. As the Bible says, there is a time to reap and a time to sow – and we don't regenerate without rest. Passive rest – much of which is sleep – works best when we know how much we individually need. Then we set up the simple conditions required to get it. Through pre-dreaming and other methods we can make sleep more regenerative and creative.

Active rest – the physical, mental, social and spiritual kinds under our own direct control – helps remake our bodies and retool our minds. By connecting our physical and spiritual selves it allows for greater unity and harmony within us – and opens us to inner capacities we never knew we had.

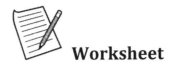 **Worksheet**

Rest is a whole lot more than sleep – but sleep itself is necessary for life.

Night

Here are a few nighttime suggestions:

- Go to the bed at the same time – every day of the week.
- Rest before sleep. Take at least 30 combined minutes to set up your sleep ritual:
- Turn down your bed.
- Put out your clothes for the next day.
- Floss and brush your teeth.
- Turn down the lights.
- Turn off your electronics – especially cell phones that ring in the night.
- Listen to soothing music.
- Read a book you should have read in high school.

If you wake up in the middle of the night and want to return to sleep –

Get out of bed inside 10 minutes – and if you're not back asleep by then –

Go to another room and read until sleepy – or listen to music.

Wake up at the same time each day.

Wake up to an alarm – it can be a well timed dog or cat; a radio program; chimes or a clock radio.

If there's sunlight out open up the drapes on waking – and stretch your muscles. Soak in that light – it can help you sleep the next night.

Your sleep was

How many hours   _____

Interrupted how many times?   _____

How restful?

(On a scale from 1-5, where 5 is excellent)   _____

Morning

Start at your work desk by visualizing your day – particularly the most important thing you want done that day. Accomplish that and you accomplish a lot.

Some time in the morning take 30-60 seconds for visualizing how you want to spend your weekend – and what you need to get done before the weekend.

Your morning included active rest techniques like

_____

_____

Afternoon

If you are so inclined – and have the chance – take a 10 to 15 minute nap. Set a timer or alarm so it won't last too long.

If you can't nap, do paradoxical relaxation for at least one minute. Use the relaxed state of concentration to revitalize you.

Go visit a work colleague or friend – if possible. Talk about something you'd really like to do in the future – preferably together.

Pre-dream – spend at least a few seconds imagining what dreams you'd like tonight.

Your afternoon included what kinds of active rest?

_____

_____

Evening

Write down before dinner the things that really bug you – and what you plan to do about them. Spend at least two to three minutes writing your answers – then read over what you've written.

Pre-dream – incorporate something you did that day into the dreams you'd like to have.

Try a moment for spiritual rest – a short prayer or moving in space – sometime between finishing your evening meal and going to sleep.

Your evening included active rest techniques like

_____

_____

If you can –

Go to bed and get up at the same times at least five times a week; feel reasonably sharp most mornings; take a minute for active rest techniques once or twice a day –

You're doing OK.

If you can –

Wake up with at least seven hours of sleep (some will need less) and feel rested (at least a 3/5 score) upon waking most days; pre-dream on occasion; write you down your worries and solutions a few times each week –

You're doing well.

If you can –

Walk after most meals; wake up feeling rested; eat primarily whole foods – both at home and when dining out; get at least 45 minutes of physical activity every day –

You're doing very well.

If you can –

Put five colors on your plate for most meals; walk for 10-15 minutes after almost every meal; stand up every hour on the job, or get moving in some other way; visit with family and friends sometime at the beginning and end of the day; feel rested when you wake –

You're doing really well.

Rest is active, and as you've seen, often exciting. Just as exercise is use of any voluntary muscle, rest can encompass numberless activities that remake and regenerate your body.

Get your mind away from thinking of rest as passive – of sitting and lying down. You want to make rest both relaxing *and* thrilling.

And social rest – what most of us call socializing – can be immensely powerful in promoting your health. Social engagement gives life meaning and purpose – along with sometimes intense pleasure.

Combine socializing with eating, moving, and resting, and you may be amazed at what you can do – regenerating body, heart and soul.

Chapter 6 - Only Connect | Socializing for Health

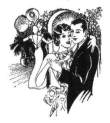

Like spending time with your friends and colleagues? You should. It's a healthy thing to do.

Most of the time, it's really healthy.

The longest-lived populations in the world – throughout the world – score high in social connection.

It's not a surprise. **We're built that way.**

And have been for a very, very long time.

Recent research has looked at primates – the species of apes that includes humans. Almost all primates have basic, similar social structures – with genes that may go back 50 million years.

We're such social animals that there are now seven billion of us on the planet – the majority packed together into cities. Despite that, most of us feel "very unique." Every one of us seems to have our own thoroughly individual consciousness.

Yet Albert Einstein, one of the most distinctive people of recent history, spoke of the "optical delusion" of individuality.

We are deeply connected in innumerable ways. We are dependent for our food, safety, energy and shelter on thousands of people we will never meet. And our different individual ecosystems interact in ways we have not even begun to study:

• About 20,000 people a year in the U.S. die from clostridium difficile, a bacterial infection caused by antibiotic use unbalancing our gut's complex ecosystem. Most or all antibiotics won't kill clostridium difficile – which is why so many people die from it. Yet 90% can be cured by transferring gut bacteria from family members to the one infected.

• When people connect with those they care about, levels of stress hormones go way down. Levels of hormones that engage connectedness and happy feelings, like oxytocin, go up.

• People in religious groups live longer and experience less depression, with much of the benefit seeming to arrive through their social connections.

• The Berkman-Syme studies of the 1970s showed that people with more social connections had fewer strokes, less heart disease, less depression; even decreased levels of tumors. Ever since, international studies across the board show *longer life and less disease the more social connections people possess.*

We are social animals. Most people consider the most important element in their lives their personal relationships.

We like people; we *love* some people. The more people we connect with, the longer we tend to live (the same appears to be true of our connections with pets).

And the better we feel. Social connection is not just healthy – it provokes perhaps the most potent pleasures we know.

Facebook World

Social connectedness is now changing – rapidly. The Internet Revolution has only begun. It will continue to change how we live, move, work, and love – for a long time.

Some changes have not been entirely beneficial. Recent studies argue that the Facebook generation may lack real empathy with others; perhaps possessing 5,000 friends does not make each of them special. Yet the ability of the Net to cheaply connect people across all time zones and geographies should be regarded as an extraordinary advantage – and not just to marketers and businesses.

There are more people than ever for you to meet out there. In many ways it's easier to meet them.

And that's what you want to do – meet them in the real world.

Because the scientific literature on social connection – *so far* – shows that face to face connection is what's truly significant for achieving real health. Meeting people "in the flesh" is very important to our lives – especially our health and our enjoyment.

Much more information gets passed when you meet people face to face than over the Net, or even when you talk to them over the phone or through Skype. Some of that information is conscious –

the way people look, their posture, the small changes of face, voice, skin.

Yet much social and biological information we pass along is not conscious. We sense someone's "body language" often without thinking about it. We feel that we like or don't like someone we've just met for reasons we can't explain – or even acknowledge.

We appear to pass pheromones, small hormones that go into the air, to each other; they change our behavior in ways of which we are not aware. The huge ecosystem inside us also modifies our bodies when we make contact with others – and not just in provoking or fighting infection. The bacteria, fungi, and viruses we exchange with other people change our immunity and our health. Kids who play more in the dirt have less asthma in later life.

The Net increases your chances for all kinds of social contacts. Yet in a world with so much connection, people complain bitterly of loneliness. Heaven is other people; so is pain.

One way to lessen that pain is to connect socially – and to maintain those connections. Almost all of us possess a social network we can use to get and become healthy.

Knowing how to access that network starts by looking where you really spend your time.

Time With Others

Look at where people spend their waking hours and the numbers are pretty stark. The big items are work, television, cellphones and computers, plus eating.

So here's how to use each to socially connect:

Connecting at Work

Social connections on the job have changed. About 15-20% of Americans who want to work can't get a job, or can get little more than occasional part-time work. Following frequent job cutbacks, many now work from home. Yet the majority of the population still finds itself making many of its human connections through jobs and school.

Recognize that the more social connections you have, the better it is for your health. When Berkman and Syme began studying social relationships in the 1970s, they mainly added up social ties and the number of organizations to which one belonged. They found the more connections people had the longer they lived.

Everything seems to count – deep, intimate relations as well as superficial ones – though with different benefits for each.

So it's a good idea to at least speak to everybody at work – no matter who they are. And here are a few things to try:

Shake hands. Don't worry about the bacteria on your fingers and palms – they will change by the hour. You can usually wash your hands quickly in a washroom nearby (or you can bring alcohol-based liquids if you're on a plane or train or bus). People feel differently about each other when they shake hands – a direct, more formal social contact has been made. You also sense more about them. Politicians and businessmen know this in their bones.

Say hello. It's good to be polite and let others know you accord them basic dignity and respect. You may not need to *say* anything. In many communities nodding the head is enough; in others it's the briefest smile. You want to acknowledge people – which provides them a chance to more fully acknowledge you.

Thank people. If they do something you appreciate, no matter how small, thank them. It may make you feel better – as well as the person to whom you've shown gratitude.

Ask questions. They can be innocuous or even appear meaningless – how you feel about today's weather. Asking questions works because many people possess a common, favorite topic – themselves. You can be extremely shy and still get far socially just by questioning people about their work, family, likes and dislikes – and asking more questions as you learn more. Generally – though certainly not always – the more you know about people, the more things you'll find to like about them. That makes it easier for you to connect.

Economic survival. Even when times are wonderful you want to know what's going on where you work. The more people you know, the *more you will know* – including facts that will affect you and your family's future.

And the more connections you have, the more potential there is for social solidarity. Companies today are creating their own social networks – because it's good business.

More connections means more – and new – ideas passed through and between divisions. More connection means people have a chance to think and act together – and cooperate. More connections also potentially promotes greater interest in the goals and opportunities of an organization or community.

Plus it means better health for you and those you know and work with. You might even find out about better deals for affordable health insurance – or a better job.

This advice goes doubly for independent contractors who have to make a living through the connections they maintain. The less your economic stress, the easier it is to be healthy – and *enjoy real health – full physical, mental, social and spiritual well-being.*

And to combine healthy effects, try to have a few walking business meetings. Go outside together – **walk and talk.**

People respond very differently to social and work connections when they're outside – especially if the weather is sunny and pleasant. Sunlight changes mood – and perspective. People may talk more openly. They express different kinds of ideas. And they can make different types of social connections, moving back and forth, talking with varied people.

Remember – sitting long is dangerous to your health. And what could be bad about walking, talking, and thinking in clear sunny air?

Connecting Through the Net

Many people have a lively social network through the Net.

Yet the complicated story of social networks and their overall health benefits is only starting to become studied – and understood. It may turn out that having Net connections alone will prove useful to your health.

It certainly pays to use the Net to create the face-to-face connections. We know those connections make people feel better – and live longer and more healthily.

So you can start "cheap meets." If you have connected with someone only through the Net, try to meet her or him in person – or if you like, meet them collectively.

In the old days when the Net was young, people who met purely via email would schedule special "live" meetings to see how the netizens they "knew" looked, talked, walked, and felt. For many the experience was a pleasant shock. For others it led to marriages and the best relationships of their lives.

It's time to revive that practice.

So invite people you find interesting to meet together. It can be at a restaurant, a park, a sports event, someone's home – or any convenient public place.

Your Internet friends can become your real world friends – and help you make connections with others. Your social network can then broaden and deepen.

Connecting Through Food

There's an old joke about the important social holidays for many different ethnic groups – "They tried to kill us; we survived. Let's eat."

Humans love to eat. We love to talk. And we really like to connect eating and talking – doing both together.

So when you eat, try to eat socially. Many families these days do not sit down as a family – even for a single meal a day.

Change that. Meals are often the place where you really find out what's going on with the people you love – and with the people you don't. Highly engaging information often gets passed from person to person when you're eating – even if it's with a tough business rival.

To socially connect through food also need not cost much out of pocket. People can meet over coffee – one reason Starbucks has done so well. You can grab a cup of tea with almost anyone – or bring it to any spot you like. The English have done this for centuries.

And you can invite people to picnic with you – bringing your own stuff to dine together – in nature. People feel better dining in a natural place – often much better – especially when there's water around.

You can always invite someone for lunch or dinner at your own home, of course. People have been doing that for longer than recorded history.

It's fun. And it's good for your health.

Connecting Through Television

For many, television is a solitary activity. You sit dumbly in front of the set, silently watching and intermittently listening – or just walk by and occasionally pay attention.

Americans keep their sets on over eight hours a day. Television can act as a soothing magnet, but it can also increase people's sense of loneliness. Some people think: if only my life could be as enjoyable or interesting as it is for folks on my favorite shows.

It does not have to work that way.

TV executives often find audience interaction is critical to their show's success. People want to feel involved.

You can obtain that interaction, too – *through your own actions.*

There's no need to watch TV alone. And unlike the movies, you can talk during TV programs.

And cajole. Joke. Satirize. Debate and laugh about what you've seen.

In olden days people provided their own entertainment. Almost everybody sang. Many played instruments. It was a major way communities connected. In much of the world, it still is.

Even with TV, such connections are possible. If you can't watch with someone else, you can connect with them over the Net – and happily comment on what you see.

Unless you're totally enthralled by what you're watching, that is.

And through this type of conversation you will learn a great deal about what others like and dislike – and how they think. Which can spur your own creativity.

Cameras are cheap in the digital age. Hundreds of millions upload to YouTube. The audience for what you say and create can be large.

Creating your own content causes you to learn new skills – and can connect you with many others. Being and feeling creative makes many people happy.

And feel and look healthier.

Summary

Humans are profoundly social animals. What most people don't know is that social connection is healthy in itself. The biological causes are not clear, but social connection is regenerative. The more the connections, the deeper, the more varied, the better off we are – at preventing heart disease, stroke and depression – and making ourselves more content, competent, and creative individuals.

And you can do so many healthy things – eat, move and rest – with others.

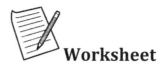 **Worksheet**

Humans are social. You can make life healthier and more fun by including others – even when you don't think what you're doing is "socializing."

Here are a few suggestions:

Morning

Walk or bike to work at least part of the way with a work colleague.

If you drive or use public transport to get to work try to join a friend or co-worker going there, too.

Say hello to people as you travel to work.

Write a note – or call – a friend, relative or work colleague first thing in the morning for some purpose – or just to let them know you're thinking of them.

Email or text someone you like but have not connected with for at least a week.

Have breakfast with a work colleague or friend.

Have a meeting with a work colleague where you're not tethered to a desk. Better, have the meeting while walking (a nice day outside makes this easier).

Your morning socialization this week included

_____

_____

Afternoon

Have lunch with a work colleague or friend.

Walk to a restaurant or park or picnic area with them – try for at least 10 minutes of walking each way.

Call a friend around lunchtime – someone you'd like to connect with.

Visit a different part of town for lunch than where you usually go – preferably through self-transport.

Have a work meeting where you and several others are walking together – preferably a different setting each time.

Stand and have a conversation – especially if you can't leave the office area. Ask them how they feel and how they're doing.

Walk to a park – for lunch or work purposes – with a colleague or friend. As you walk, talk about the food – how it's grown, where it comes from, what information it gives your body.

Go visit a work colleague – or neighbor – for at least two to three minutes, and see if there's something you can do together at a later time. Ask about their health. Shake their hand as you meet, or as you leave.

Your afternoon socialization included

_____

_____

Evening

Eat with your family – even if you have a hundred excuses not to.

Get everyone possible to help with shopping, cooking, and cleaning up after the meal.

Stroll or walk with family or friends after dining for at least 10 to 15 minutes.

Watch TV with someone else. Use a stepper part of the time if you can but still talk – commenting and hopefully joking about what you're watching.

Have a dinner party at least once a month; inviting relatives, friends, or people from work – cooking only whole foods.

Get the family to plan vegetarian meals for the next week – discussing it at the supper table – and as you walk afterwards.

Call up, email or text an old friend you have not spoken to for at least a month.

Plan a trip with people you love.

Your evening socialization involved

_____

_____

If you can –

Talk to family and friends a couple of times a day; eat with your family at least once a day; walk with friends or families some days –

You're doing OK.

If you can –

Talk to family and friends at different times of day; do active rest techniques – like preparing a meal – with family and friends once a day; connect with your friends at least once a week, face to face or electronically; walk with family, friends or colleagues at least once a week; get in at least 30 minutes of some kind of physical activity most days –

You're doing well.

If you can –

Eat with work colleagues and walk to lunch and back; use self-transport to get to work; walk after most meals; take several times a day to actively rest – pre-dream, do visualizations or PR; get 45 minutes of some kind of physical activity each day; obtain seven hours of rest most every night and wake feeling refreshed –

You're doing very well.

If you can –

Wake up feeling sharp; move after most every meal; have a pattern to the day where you eat and rest and move at scheduled times; schedule at least two times each week to just socialize with family and friends; use self-transport every chance you can; connect with something larger than oneself –

You're doing really well.

And you're starting to put things together – which makes them really count.

Because putting these basic activities together greatly helps you regenerate. The body works as a system. And you can then regenerate your body more the way you want – and become more of what you wish to become.

Regeneration is a different paradigm – the real way your body works to remake itself – and learn.

To learn more – read on.

Chapter 7 - The Promise of Regeneration

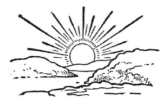

Know what regenerates your body and you can make a new you.

That's what this book is about.

The message can be simplified to this: use your body the way it's built.

Use the technology that evolution gives you and you can remake yourself. Walking rather than sitting changes your brain, your waistline, and your mood. Cooking whole foods rather than ordering pizza changes guts, brains, arteries – and can dramatically shift your relationship with the environment. Visiting friends can entertain, inspire, make you happier and more knowledgeable – and prevent Alzheimer's disease and heart attacks.

Put them all together and the results improve again.

Knowing how to regenerate yourself can keep you healthy – get you healthy – and make you more vibrant, resilient, and alive. Alive to the world inside – and the world beyond.

Everything you do counts – everything changes your inner information flow second by second. The simplest acts help remake your body, your mood, your attitude, and your future.

Not to mention saving enormous amounts of healthcare dollars.

Because we are what we do – and what we do is what we become.

Yet most of us don't see this amazing process. In part that's because we mainly remake and replace ourselves internally, hidden from view.

The "miracle" of regenerating yourself the way you like can happen because most of your body is replaced – from the inside out – within a few weeks. **We see our hair grow; our nails grow – but not our quickly developing brain.** A python can double the size of its inner organs – heart, lungs, and spleen – within 24 hours.

Do you see your heart mainly replaced within three days? No. Do you see your brain rewire itself every night? No. Do you see your immune system creating billions of new antibodies to confront new invaders? No.

Yet what we don't see is *far vaster* than what we do. We regenerate ourselves rapidly and powerfully – from within. The python gets bigger. Our brains and bodies get smarter.

Regeneration – the Real Aim

Regeneration is the process by which your body survives. We're not machines – we're organisms.

Don't think of your body as a machine. Machines fall apart. We remake ourselves – continually. That's how we stay alive. And we use our constituent parts so quickly we constantly need to make new ones.

And we're never the same – not even from moment to moment. If we were machines – like cars or boats or toasters – we'd look and act the same all our lives.

And never be born, grow up, mature, adapt, learn, experience and age. Or know true joy.

We don't see how quickly we replace ourselves – or how immense and complete are the changes within.

But change they do. **The awesome speed of those changes gives us the chance to use our best technology – our bodies – to become what we want to become.**

Think of it this way – if most of a human body is remade inside a month, can't I do a lot to remake myself?

Life is Fast

Your gut lining is replaced within a couple of days – completely. You have entirely new skin on your face within two weeks – all new cells. Yet the microscopic processes of your body – like cell repair – are *far more rapid.* They remake most everything inside long before your cells may divide and reproduce. You rapidly remake yourself from the inside out.

Much of the hard work of that regeneration is performed by proteins. Proteins create much of cell communication. They pass information, make and modify almost all living chemicals, produce and become bone and sinew. Even enzymes are proteins, speeding the chemistry of life.

How fast do proteins work? Estimates are there are a billion protein-protein interactions – information events – every second.

Per cell.

You have 10 trillion human cells.

No wonder most proteins last only hours to days. Our energy supplies – like glucose and fats – are modified even more quickly. Most are used and re-formed within seconds to minutes.

Even our relatively stable DNA is modified thousands of times an hour. It has to repair itself with extreme accuracy – or undergo potentially fatal mutation.

Life is fast – superfast. We use up materials and energy very quickly. They all have to be replaced.

This happens partly because of the intensely competitive environment we live in. Remember – **you are a complex ecosystem**. You may have 10 trillion human cells – but there are 100 trillion bacteria in your gut alone. Many might become pathogens if we did not control them.

That immune challenge alone is a gigantic, never-finished job. The information processing, energy and materials required are enormous.

To understand how big the job is let's look at just one single virus – among the thousands of different types of organisms living inside us. Hepatitis B is one of the leading global causes of cancer and death.

When we get a hepatitis B infection the virus will normally reproduce 100 billion copies.

In one day.

Each copy can then make a new virus – potentially mutated to confuse our immune system – *inside four hours.*

And the massive task of fighting off that infection is not the immune system's sole critical job. If our body doesn't *learn* during the time we root out infections – figuring out which organisms are OK and which are not, understanding how to destroy or at least control the malefactors – we don't survive.

Regeneration doesn't just quickly remake our bodies. Regeneration changes how we learn – *and how we turn out.*

Because we get better. Smarter. Better adapted. More efficient.

Our bodies never stop learning, not until we ourselves end –

Our immune system uses directed hypermutation to create new antibodies to fight off infection.

Consider what happens after we slip crossing a crooked step. We may lose a few ligament and muscle cells. Yet the new ones that grow in should prove better suited for what comes next.

Our brain's three-dimensional tracking system instantly resets with every move we make. We learn more quickly and directly exactly where we are – and how to move most effectively. That changes the regrowth of our muscles and limbs – all through the day. They will be remade differently – with much of that remaking occurring in sleep.

Our eyes look around us and remember the environment – its perils and pleasures – making new memories.

We are always creating new knowledge. That new knowledge remakes us – an ongoing process *that does not stop.* It's a process of re-creation that makes us wiser, more capable of dealing with the new stresses that assault us every day.

We can also use that new knowledge to keep and make us healthier.

Using Evolution to Innovate You

Evolution is used against you every day. Environmental scarcity gave you a body constructed to survive chronic intermittent starvation. Salt, sugar, and fat were hard to find – so you crave them all. Humans became upright and extraordinarily efficient walking machines that marched across the Earth, from the North to the South Poles. We scaled Mt. Everest and all the highest peaks.

Internal cell receptors evolved to control pain and exertion and reward reproduction and ingesting sweet, starvation-stopping food.

Now those evolutionary quirks are used to make money – lots of money.

Pain and pleasure receptors can be stimulated and programmed by heroin and cocaine – so efficient at making us forget everything that they destroy innumerable lives. The same brain reward circuitry also responds to magnificent confections like vanilla chocolate chip milkshakes – whose effects on the brain mirror cocaine. Bodies built to run and dance watch *others* run and dance – on TV and the Net. When we gain weight our highly evolved starvation-fighting bodies fight weight loss – all the way down. We still feel hungry even when our weight has dropped to "normal."

Here's a better idea: use all that evolutionary machinery to make you look better, feel great, work more effectively and have more fun. And potentially last longer.

That's what you've been learning in this book.

A little knowledge goes a long way:

Food – eating the whole foods your body is built for is easier, cheaper, more nutritious, educational and entertaining. Eating the regenerative way will help make you light, able, and nimble. An added plus – emphasizing whole foods is better for the whole planet.

All voluntary muscle activity can become effective exercise. Your body is a walking machine that exults in being used. And you can use your body well in almost any imaginable environment – work, home, school, even cars or airplanes. Moving your body naturally, doing the cooking and cleaning, visiting your co-workers and neighbors does not require a gym – *it doesn't require one red cent*. And it can improve your looks *and* save your life.

Rest has been the giant elephant in the room, unappreciated and neglected. Yet it is a giant force that can revitalize you, amuse you – and help you control your weight and avoid chronic disease.

Socializing is not just fun. It's what much of your body and brain are built for. It's a great way to connect – be entertained – find love – and discover meaning. It makes life worthwhile, and can motivate you to fulfill yourself – and exceed all expectations. It can also inspire you to do the simple actions that regenerate your body and make you healthier.

You can get evolution to work for you by doing the most ordinary things in the world. The whole shooting match works far better when you put those ordinary actions together.

Make it into a system and the system will work for you – every second of the day.

Synergy

Your body's amazing inner technology works incredibly well. It works that much better when you coordinate basic activities.

Synergy means effects are more than additive when put together.

Evolution knows those facts well. To get the biggest bang for your buck it takes critical processes – like food gathering and energy production – and meshes them into a system.

That's exactly what you want to do for yourself, family, friends and community.

Food is about a lot more than calories. Move before a meal and you may increase your metabolism – a little. But move *after* a meal and you change your basic metabolism – making it easier to control weight and slim your waistline. You can remake white fat into brown – changing belly fat, too. You can change the speed and effectiveness of cell recycling – making regeneration easier.

No one says you need to cook alone – or buy food by yourself. Socializing is what we're built to do. It's great fun when we cook, eat, and carouse together.

Of course you can follow a meal with a social stroll. A simple walk can improve your immune system, alert your mind – and, especially when timed in the morning, make it easier for you to sleep that night.

Walking with a friend to lunch or dinner will, after only 20-30 minutes, help you produce new brain cells. They will grow up in memory areas – as you sleep. And you'll quickly be using them to remember and improve memory.

Walking with a relative or colleague does more than grow relationships. It grows your brain. That little walk will help you fight off infection – decrease your risk of heart attack, cancer, and stroke – and perhaps provide sunlight that improves mood and fights off the blues.

So look at the basics – food, activity, rest, socializing. They all support each other. They all make the others work better. They can all make your day more fun.

Put them together and they help regenerate you.

They can also save you money – while they extend your life. How else do Asian American women on Long Island expect to last more than 95 years?

What's one easy way to put them together? Try this – just remember three letters – **FAR. They stand for Food, Activity, and Rest.**

One simple, easy system is to do one of them followed by the next – throughout the daytime. You eat, you move, you rest.

And you can socialize as you eat, move, and rest – increasing the benefits.

The **FAR** system works even better if you eat, move, rest and socialize according to your own personal schedule. The improvement occurs because your body is built on time.

Remember – **Time rules life.**

Put food, activity, rest and socializing into a regular, scheduled pattern and you can achieve real synergy. You then create your own simple, individual daily program that can maximize efficiency, energy, healthiness and potential longevity.

The system works well for the simplest reason – we're built that way. We remake ourselves every moment of our lives. **Regeneration is what we do to stay alive – and thrive. And regeneration works by getting the right information at the right times.**

Regeneration-Information-Health – a New Health Paradigm

It's time for you – and medical care – to move past the machine model of the body. Most of us think of our bodies as machines. Usually we compare our bodies with the most complicated machines we know. In the 19th century bodies were compared with steam engines.

Now we conceive of the human body as similar to a computer. The brain is our software, the rest of our body hardware.

That approach is simple and common. *And so very wrong.*

Your body is greater than any computer, any machine. You update every second. You learn enormous amounts every fraction of a second.

And most of that learning is unconscious.

Think of driving a car – or texting on a cell phone. Do you verbally tell yourself: "turn the steering wheel 16 degrees in the next quarter second to avoid that darting squirrel moving at a 37 degree angle to the midline?"

Of course not. All that is the work of implicit memory.

And the immense work of your immune system, your gut, and your muscles? Most of that is much farther from conscious thought than the implicit memory that lets you drive a car or ride a bicycle.

Yet that incredible mass of instant information is constantly used to repair, renew and regenerate you. The work is done with extraordinary speed. **You always change – you never stop learning.**

No machine can do that.

Please don't think of yourself as a machine. Your capacities are vastly greater. You're an organism. You're alive. You're conscious.

And what you and every organism on the planet does is process information.

Think of it this way:

You go to a concert of Cold Play – or Rihanna. Later you see the same concert as an online video. The pixels you see on the screen exist because a video machine processed visual and auditory information into individual bits. They can be sent anywhere on the Net.

But does that video capture *everything* you experienced? The smells and sights – the songs you heard in your head before they played – the memories of other concerts? Does it include the way your ears recoiled when you stood too close to a speaker – or the feeling in the pit of your stomach at the end of a song? Can that video define and describe all the people you saw and felt moving through the crowd?

And can a video even start to define all the unconscious information of that concert – how your immune system reacted to the thousands of other people and their viruses and bacteria – what happened to your muscles and joints when you nearly tripped on a soda bottle – the way the light show reverberated inside your brain, dazzling you – and changing your body's inner clocks?

No way.

The amount of information your body and brain take in with every breath is vastly, vastly greater than anything in any video. All that vast information keeps your body learning – every second of your life. It's the type of learning that keeps you alive – and physically renews you.

Give your body the right information – for how you eat, move, rest and socialize – and it will learn better, remake itself better, regenerate itself more effectively.

And make you more of what you want to become.

Regeneration is how your body works. Information processing is how it gets the job done. Give your body the right information and you can experience real health – physical, mental, social and spiritual well being.

The Swedish novelist Lars Gustafsson wrote, "we begin again – we never give up."

Your body does not give up – not until the very end. It remakes itself, updates itself, renews itself – every moment you're alive. The information that comes with how you eat, move, rest and socialize can change nearly everything – especially when you combine those actions together. Many of us have the power to make our bodies thrive beyond our hopes.

Let this book help you take back your body – and take control over your health.

Doing What's Needed

Getting your body to regenerate is not hard – once you know what to do. All the little things count.

Put them together and they count even more.

Walking 15 minutes more each week can change your waistline *and* help clean your arteries. Replacing a processed starch with a vegetable once a week can help remake your brain and gut. Calling up an old friend both revives and remakes old memories. It can give you a shot at more pleasure, more love – and a greater understanding of who and what you are.

Your health is about your resilience – your ability to meet and overcome the new stresses of every day. Your real health – your physical, mental, social and spiritual well-being – includes your ability to learn and create. You want to increase your capacity to do new things, to imagine new ways, to produce new forms, to make yourself more what you wish to become.

The process provides its own reward. It can give you new enjoyments and adventures each day.

And along the way you can feel better, look better, and think more clearly and perceptively.

Improving your health is merely a healthy byproduct to a regenerative life – a life where you experience more, feel more, and create new and deeper meanings. That form of expansive, exuberant real health is possible – when you know how to regenerate your body.

The good stuff adds up.

Individually we possess the capacity to remake and regenerate our bodies and lives.

Our health care system does not.

Real National Health

Greece and the American health care system have a lot in common.

As of this writing, Greece has technically defaulted on its national debt. The reason – it borrowed a lot more money than it produced.

Public sector workers made more than those in private industry – and often did not show up for work. Not paying taxes was a matter of principle. Tax collectors expected bribes – particularly in election years.

The money went out. Not enough came in. There's scant chance that Greece can eventually grow its way out of its remaining debt. The cascading results have produced an international financial crisis that may eventually provoke a body blow to the world economy.

America cannot grow fast enough to pay its future health care costs.

Between 1960 and 1997 American health care costs increased by 9.4% each year. Economic growth was a fraction of that. That's why health care cost 5% of our total economic product in 1972, and 17% today. That's how American health care alone became as big as the economy of France.

The American economy is hardly growing – but our elderly population is rapidly rising. The fastest growing segment in the population – those over 85. Their health care costs are high. Plus there's annual inflation *and* the increased costs of medical technology advances. Add in the increasing size of the general population. The peak baby boomer birth year was 1957. As boomers increase in age, so do their health costs.

Where will that money come from? That's going to be your job.

How much can you pay? How much have you got?

Even those with health insurance can expect more of what I see every day – bills for $4,000 for tests an insurer originally agreed to – but now refuses to pay. A $6,000 diagnostic bill no one is willing to accept.

Even people with "great" insurance will be caught holding the bag. Medical bankruptcies will increase.

As the pie shrinks economic wars will break out over who gets to keep the money. That most of the developed world does a better job for half the cost – and that their methods can be copied – will probably not enter the political debate. The media will report what they claim interests viewers, but you will mainly hear what they are paid to report. Insurance companies, device companies, Big Pharma, hospitals and medical providers (which means me) will all try to keep our share. Expect the big boys to get the cash first.

Yet health care disaster is not inevitable. Real national health is much more important than health care. We should pay attention to three propositions:

1. Health is the goal of health care. Health is what counts. If we spent our effort on improving our health – or just possessed a mixed health care system like that of Germany – we could save well over a trillion dollars every year. Think of what that money could do to reduce indebtedness – and to increase economic competitiveness.

2. A healthy economy requires a healthy population. Healthier people work more effectively. We also need to recognize that our food policies greatly affect our health. A future America where three in 10 is diabetic is a health and economic catastrophe.

3. A healthy population requires a healthy environment – live in a toxic place and you'll get sick.

Sadly we cannot expect our political and economic leadership to do the right thing. Nuclear reactors can disintegrate slowly – or quickly. Our housing crisis will just be practice for the coming health care meltdown.

You need to protect yourself. Your best insurance remains and will remain keeping yourself healthy, vibrant, and well. You do that by efficiently regenerating your body and brain.

And you get there by investing in frugal innovation – for and by yourself. You get to use and improve the best technology available to you – your human body. Give that body the right information and it can remake itself right.

For what are disease and aging but failures of regeneration? That should be the new health paradigm – to naturally and simply help everyone **regenerate as effectively as we are capable**. Illness is not a breakdown of the "machine." Illness is not regenerating correctly.

Yet with time, all of us will find that our regeneration eventually fails. As my grandmother said, nobody gets out of this life alive.

So what can you do when you get sick? In these crazy times, how to navigate our broken health care system is a huge topic. But the next chapter gives you some basic guidelines on what paths you can take – even when you lack individual resources.

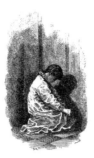

Obtaining Health Care When You Get Sick

First and foremost, stay well. Sadly, even for the healthiest people regeneration is never perfect. It's normal that at some point you will get sick with something far worse than a cold or a sprained muscle.

If you're really ill and lack health insurance, going to a hospital or ER may prove scary. Unfortunately, with some exceptions, you should expect to get ripped off.

Hospitals usually charge the uninsured *what they can't get from the insured.* That means every dime they can. Don't expect their numbers to be logical or believable – just legally enforceable.

So the first order of business is to stay healthy – one reason you've read this short book. The next order of business is to monitor yourself for common illnesses (see below).

So what do you do if struck with an illness that simply has to be treated?

You negotiate.

Negotiation is generally easier with doctors than hospitals. Tell a doctor what you want. Then she can tell you a figure of what that will cost. If it's in cash, she'll probably give you a discount.

GPs are generally reasonable – figuring their cost in time spent, plus whatever materials they need. Not infrequently, the materials are the most expensive item.

Hospitals have giant bureaucracies and cost structures that have evolved rather like medieval legal codes. Soon the number of disease/diagnostic codes will reach 140,000 – crazy! Often hospitals don't know or can't figure out what they should charge you for a service. They themselves can receive different payments from virtually every vendor, and those can change by the week.

So when negotiating with hospitals or clinics, try to make a deal. If you need an operation and there's no other way, make offers and counter-offers. People prefer receiving some money to none.

Or you can go to sources that don't cost at all.

Cheap Health Providers

County health departments are supposed to protect the public health. If you have no insurance – and no money – some will pay for a lot of care. Sadly, others will cover practically nothing – and as budgets bite, less and less.

The best way to find out what health departments do provide is to **show up and ask.** You can certainly call first – but what they say on the phone may not be true when you arrive.

The same is true of county hospitals. Many by law are supposed to take care of you no matter what – if you have an emergency.

Their definition of emergency is, of course, *very* variable – even elastic. So are their definitions of "treatment" and "stabilization." Most hospitals operate these days as if they were for-profit institutions – regardless of what it says on the entrance.

There are also large regional differences. New York City has long been a mecca for those seeking health care without the ability to pay. Much of my training was at such hospitals.

Still, the money for many public institutions is fast disappearing – even though the eventual costs to the country – and taxpayers – will prove much higher.

Other places to look for care include:

Free clinics – usually operated by county hospitals, federal and state agencies, or churches.

Senior centers – lots of docs are fed up with health care and retiring – but do not want to stop using their skills. Senior care centers often have a group of docs around who will try and help you.

Schools – many kids will get physicals through public schools – especially when sport seasons begin.

Surprisingly, life insurance companies often provide a physical to those trying to obtain life insurance – free of charge. Getting your results may take some doing, though.

Monitoring Your Health When Asymptomatic

Does everybody need a yearly physical? No. If you're without any medical symptoms and under 50, and of course, don't smoke, some public health physicians would argue you don't need do much beyond the simple monitoring discussed below. If you do have symptoms, county health departments, or GPs with whom you negotiate a price, may provide what you need.

However, physicals every few years may make sense for those undergoing the increasing difficulties of modern life. And you yourself should *at least* look yearly at some basic measures:

Blood Pressure

Blood pressure should be monitored from childhood on. In adults, you will get different academic answers as to what level requires treatment. Some public health experts think that, for adults, a blood pressure of 160/90 is a clarion call for major lifestyle changes and medication. Other national organizations argue anything above 120/80 is too high. Some might split the difference at 140/90. However, recognize that lower blood pressure is better – down to a quite low level indeed. Also recognize blood pressure naturally varies 15% by time of day, going higher as the afternoon and evening approach.

You can get your blood pressure taken at supermarkets and health clubs. However, automatic machines are often uncalibrated – and frequently inaccurate.

The County Health Department can help here. Most free clinics will quickly oblige a request to take your pressure.

And regular, accurate blood pressure cuffs can be had – with stethoscope – for around $20-$30. It's not hard to learn to take your blood pressure – and families can share around a blood pressure cuff.

Weight

Supermarket scales will suffice here – though many of you have your own scale. If you're an adult and your weight is going up more than 2-3% a year, it's time to look very carefully at what you eat, how you move, and when and how you rest. Remember – the bigger you are, the harder it is to lose weight.

Diabetes

A urine dipstick can be bought and used annually. Kits of 100 go for around $20-$35. In a population where 30 percent of us may become diabetic, it's well worth the outlay.

Depression

Depression is becoming almost epidemic in America. If you're uninterested, tired, listless, unable to sleep, can't concentrate, and simply don't enjoy what you used to enjoy, you may be joining a very large number of depressed Americans.

Recognize that anti-depressants have been oversold – at least for treating depression – as opposed to preventing it. The British treat depression with group walks in the woods. The Dutch send people to work on farms. Higher levels of physical activity, light, and social support can all help ward off depression – as can many of the suggestions in this book.

Will diet make a big difference? Depressives eat very strangely – generally overemphasizing sugar, salt and fat. However, there's no good evidence so far that healthy diets – on their own – treat clinical depression. Instead, many psychotherapies can be applied inexpensively. Some are now being tried over the Net.

Teeth

Dental health is crucial to overall health. Please try to floss and brush twice a day; Sonicare is my favorite toothbrush for fighting periodontal disease, which can cause generalized inflammation and worsen heart disease. Most of us will need to follow up with dentists every two years – at the minimum.

Look at dental care prices. Now you have an idea of what health care may cost you in the future.

Vaccines

Vaccination is certainly a must for children. Some vaccines, like flu shots and pneumococcal vaccine, certainly help older folks.

Lipids (cholesterol – HDL and LDL)

Statins are now mainly generic and can be highly effective drugs – lowering the risk of death from a major killer, cardiovascular disease – and perhaps other diseases. But present guidelines argue that you only use statins when you have clear and present cardiac risk factors – like high cholesterol. Unfortunately, statins can produce lots of side effects – including horrible ones.

County health departments and free health clinics will often cover simple chemical tests. Commercial labs vary. Some will negotiate far more readily than others.

Still, you should be able to get lipids testing for less than $10.

One advantage of using health departments and free clinics is that they will usually explain to you what the results mean. Please don't just look at absolute numbers. Labs vary dramatically in what is considered normal or abnormal, depending on their own quite variable equipment.

Remember, *numbers are just that* – numbers. Tests can be done incorrectly. Results may prove inaccurate. Statistically, do enough tests and abnormalities will show up – expect that.

Which means it pays to not have too many tests – especially the kind given at "free screenings." Such screening programs want your future business – and may not provide the most accurate results. Though most health clinics will be entirely honest in providing tests they think accurate, false positives are very common – and can prove lucrative. In his excellent book **"Overdiagnosed"**, internist H. Gilbert Welch and co-authors explain that 86% of otherwise asymptomatic people given "whole body CT scans" had at least one "abnormality." The average number of abnormalities per person was nearly three.

Which of course means you need more tests to "understand" those abnormalities.

Cancer Screening Tests - PSA and Mammography

Cancer screening is controversial and complex – with guidelines for use that can change by the month.

The government is now almost discouraging PSA testing for prostate cancer. Newer studies show 30-100 people getting treated for each individual "helped" – and with high risks of urinary incontinence and sexual impotence for those treated.

Mammography looks like it is helpful overall – but probably does not add much if you examine your breasts monthly, feeling for lumps.

Rather few asymptomatic women or men seem to be aided by cancer screening before the age of 50 – or if older than 75.

So remember – **test enough and you'll find something – particularly more tests.** Always know the purpose of any medical test – and whether the ensuing treatment will usefully affect your life.

So do check your weight, teeth, blood pressure, lipids and diabetes status – as they all affect your long-term health.

What really changes things is knowing what *you* can do – all by yourself – to regenerate your body.

Because that can lead you to real health – a full sense of well-being.

And let you stay out of the hospital.

Made in the USA
Lexington, KY
21 July 2017